Bent Leg Raise & PNF Exercise in Improving Hamstring Muscle Performance

Kshtrashal Singh
Yu Chye Wah
H'ng Ming Zhan

Bent Leg Raise & PNF Exercise in Improving Hamstring Muscle Performance

ELIVA PRESS

ISBN: 978-99993-4-599-6

Cover Design: Eliva Press
Cover Image: www.ingimage.com
Email: info@elivapress.com
Website: www.elivapress.com

This Eliva Press imprint is published by the registered company Eliva Press Global Ltd. part of Eliva Press S.R.L. Publishing Group

The registered company address is: Pope Hennessy Street Level 2, Hennessy Tower Port Louis, Mauritius
Eliva Press S.R.L. Publishing Group legal address is: Bd. Cuza-Voda 1/4 of. 21, Chisinau, Moldova, Europe

Effectiveness of Mulligan Bent Leg Raise Versus PNF Hold-Relax Exercise in Improving Hamstring Range of Motion and Muscle Performance: A Randomized Controlled Trial.

INTRODUCTION

1.1 Background of Study

Hamstring flexibility and muscle performance are important in functional mobility regarding daily activities, physical health at large, and athletic performances. Gracile movement, postural stability, and comfortable execution of basic activities such as walking, bending, or sitting are all facilitated by hamstring flexibility in normal individuals. Similarly, for athletes, hamstring flexibility is important in performance enhancement and reduction in the risk of sustaining a sports-related injury. Both groups benefit from the maintenance of an optimal hamstring ROM because tight or inflexible hamstrings eventually cause compensatory movement patterns, postural imbalances, and increased susceptibility to musculoskeletal issues. While athletes rely on their hamstring function for high-intensity activities like running and jumping, these same principles of flexibility and strength directly influence the quality of life and long-term mobility in non-athletic populations. (Claudino et al., 2021).

Dysfunctions about hamstring flexibility, including reduced ROM and tightness, may negatively impact posture and reduce efficiency in lower limb mechanics. These dysfunctions commonly result in compensatory movement patterns that increase injury risk and diminish physical performance. Reduced ROM of the hamstrings has been associated with strength production and neuromuscular efficiency deficits. Interventions such as myofascial release have been shown to significantly improve hamstring range of motion and flexibility. It also effectively reduces tightness and enhances the overall function of the muscle. These techniques can resolve fascial restrictions and increase muscle elasticity which can provide advantages in both clinical contexts and athletic performance settings (Spinoso et al., 2022).

Movement Efficiency and Hamstring Flexibility

An individual effortlessly gliding through a morning run exemplifies the ideal state of movement efficiency, where muscular coordination, flexibility, and strength work in perfect harmony. However, achieving such fluid motion is often hindered by musculoskeletal restrictions, among which hamstring tightness is one of the most prevalent factors limiting lower limb mobility. Restricted hamstring flexibility not only affects athletic performance but also has broader implications for posture, movement mechanics, and injury risk.

The hamstrings are a group of three muscles: biceps femoris, semitendinosus, and semimembranosus. This group of muscles spans the back of the thigh and plays a pivotal role in hip extension, knee flexion, and dynamic stabilization. These muscles act in synergy with the gluteal and lower back musculature to facilitate fundamental movements such as walking, running, squatting, and jumping. However, when the hamstrings become stiff or shortened, they limit the functional range of motion (ROM), which subsequently alters biomechanical efficiency and increases the likelihood of injury. Recent evidence also shows that reduced hamstring flexibility contributes to lumbar dysfunction and low back pain, and targeted interventions such as PNF stretching can improve ROM and functional outcomes in this population (Effectiveness of PNF Stretching in Hamstring Tightness with Low Back Pain Population, 2024).

Hamstring tightness is not confined to a specific group; it is observed in both sedentary individuals and high-performance athletes. Among sedentary populations, prolonged sitting leads to adaptive muscle shortening, resulting in compromised hip mobility and lumbar spine strain. Conversely, athletes frequently experience hamstring stiffness due to high eccentric loading, sprint mechanics, and repetitive high-impact movements. These activities will cause muscle fatigue, microtrauma, and a greater risk of strain injuries. Despite its high prevalence, hamstring tightness is often overlooked until it manifests as pain, functional limitations, or movement restrictions.

Understanding Hamstring Tightness: Mechanisms and Classifications

Hamstring tightness is characterized by a reduction in muscle extensibility, leading to a limited range of motion (ROM), discomfort, and compensatory movement adaptations. Clinically, it is assessed through restricted hip flexion ROM during a straight leg raise (SLR) test or a reduced knee extension angle when sitting with an extended leg (Dabhi, 2023). Hamstring tightness can be classified into two primary categories based on its onset and underlying causes: acute tightness and chronic tightness.

Acute hamstring tightness arises temporarily due to muscle fatigue, overuse, or lack of post-exercise stretching. This often happens after intense workouts where the hamstrings experience increased passive stiffness due to the metabolic byproducts accumulating within muscle fibers. On the other hand, chronic hamstring tightness develops gradually due to habitual poor posture, neuromuscular imbalances, and structural adaptations. This is commonly observed in individuals with a history of lower back dysfunction, anterior pelvic tilt, or muscle dominance imbalances which usually happen in most of the common individuals.

The key symptoms of hamstring tightness include reduced hip flexion ROM which can impair everyday movements such as deep squatting or stair climbing. This will usually cause a pulling sensation or discomfort in the posterior thigh and often accompanies stretching or dynamic movements. Additionally, individuals with tight hamstrings frequently adopt compensatory movement strategies such as excessive lumbar flexion during forward bending which eventually increases their risk of lower back pain. Functional movement such as inefficiencies resulting from hamstring tightness leads to a suboptimal force that transmits during activities such as sprinting and agility-based sports. Given its widespread impact across all age groups and activity levels. This address states that targeted interventions for hamstring tightness are essential for maintaining musculoskeletal health (Tatlıcı et al., 2021).

The Role of Hamstring Flexibility in Human Movement

Hamstring flexibility is fundamental to postural control, functional movement, athletic performance and rehabilitation. Postural control, and spinal alignment are directly influenced by hamstring extensibility as tight hamstrings contribute to posterior pelvic tilt which disrupts lumbar spine curvature and increases the risk of chronic lower back pain. Research indicates that individuals with tight hamstrings show a greater tendency toward lumbar flexion compensation which increases stress on the intervertebral discs over time and will eventually lead to degenerative changes over time (Encarnación-Martínez A, 2023). From a biomechanical perspective, hamstring flexibility plays a vital role in functional movement, and gait mechanics. The efficiency of lower limb coordination requires adequate hamstring extensibility as limited ROM has been associated with shortened stride length, increased metabolic cost of movement and inefficient shock absorption. These restrictions not only impair daily locomotion but also affect sports performance, particularly in movements requiring speed and agility.

In the context of athletic performance and injury prevention, optimal hamstring flexibility is essential for executing explosive movements, quick deceleration, and rapid directional changes. Studies have established that reduction of hamstring ROM increases risk for muscle strains, anterior cruciate ligament (ACL) injuries, and chronic tendinopathies. Conversely, improving hamstring flexibility enhances sprint efficiency, acceleration forces, and power output, leading to better athletic outcomes. This makes flexibility training a critical component of sports conditioning programs(Wan X, 2017).

Additionally, hamstring flexibility plays a key role in rehabilitation and recovery. Many post-injury rehabilitation protocols emphasize the restoration of hamstring flexibility to prevent recurrent strains and functional impairments. Physiotherapists frequently incorporate dynamic stretching, proprioceptive neuromuscular facilitation and Mulligan techniques to restore neuromuscular control and tissue elasticity. These techniques aim to improve ROM while minimizing the risk of overstretching-induced injuries, making them valuable tools in clinical settings(Kim G, 2018).

Prevalence and Risk Factors of Hamstring Tightness

Hamstring tightness is common among various populations, with multiple risk factors contributing to its development. Sedentary behavior is a primary cause, as individuals who sit for prolonged periods, particularly more than six hours per day, are significantly more likely to develop hamstring tightness due to sustained muscle shortening and reduced neuromuscular activation(Patel P, 2023).

Muscle imbalances also contribute to hamstring tightness, particularly among athletes who exhibit a quadriceps-dominant movement pattern. This imbalance creates excessive anterior chain loading, which leads to increased hamstring stiffness and reduced knee joint stability (Croisier JL, 2008). Similarly, improper training methods, such as inadequate warm-ups and a lack of post-exercise stretching, accelerate the accumulation of muscle stiffness over time.

Furthermore, aging and genetic factors influence hamstring flexibility, as muscle elasticity naturally declines with age. As individuals grow older, collagen cross-linking increases within connective tissues, reducing muscle compliance and making flexibility training crucial for maintaining functional mobility. Genetic predisposition may also play a role, as some individuals inherently possess stiffer muscle-tendon units, requiring more targeted interventions to maintain optimal flexibility levels(Pratt J, 2019).

Link to the Study: Why Compare Manual Therapy Techniques?

Given the far-reaching impact of hamstring flexibility on movement and injury risk, physiotherapists continuously seek effective intervention strategies to enhance ROM and muscle performance. This study compares two widely used manual therapy techniques:

1. Mulligan Bent Leg Raise (BLR): This technique utilizes joint mobilization and active movement to enhance hamstring flexibility and neuromuscular function.
2. PNF Hold-Relax with Agonist Contraction (HR-AC): This method incorporates isometric contraction followed by passive stretching, leveraging neuromuscular inhibition principles to improve ROM

Despite the widespread use of both techniques, limited comparative research exists on their immediate effects on hamstring flexibility and muscle performance. By filling this research gap, the present study aims to provide evidence-based awareness of the efficacy of Mulligan BLR and PNF HR-AC in enhancing ROM, improving hamstring muscle strength, and optimizing neuromuscular control.

1.2: The Anatomy and Biomechanics of the Hamstrings

Introduction to the Hamstring Muscle Group

A key component of human movement, postural stability, and injury prevention is the hamstring muscle which is found in the thigh's posterior compartment. The biceps femoris, semitendinosus, and semimembranosus are the three components of this muscle. Lower limb stability, hip extension, and knee flexion are all controlled by this muscle group. The hamstrings are crucial for mobility and biomechanical efficiency in high-performance sports motions like sprinting, jumping and quick direction changes as well as in daily tasks like walking, climbing stairs, and getting out of a seated posture. The hamstrings undergo significant mechanical loads because of their dual-joint function, especially during eccentric loading during deceleration movements. The structure of the hamstring makes them extremely vulnerable to muscular imbalances and tightness which increase the risk of strain injuries, and reduce movement efficiency, especially in physically active people. Optimizing rehabilitation treatments and injury prevention procedures requires a deeper understanding of their anatomical structure, biomechanical function, and common dysfunctions.

Anatomical Structure of the Hamstrings

The hamstrings originate from the ischial tuberosity of the pelvis and insert at different locations along the tibia and fibula which allows them to act across both the hip and knee joints. This biarticular nature of the joint enables them to contribute to both hip and knee movements but also increases their susceptibility to overuse and strain injuries. The biceps femoris, positioned laterally, and consists of two heads: the long head which originates from the ischial tuberosity, and the short head that uniquely originates from the linea aspera of the femur. Unlike the other two hamstring muscles, the short head does not cross the hip joint making it function exclusively at the knee. Both heads converge to insert at the head of the fibula facilitating knee flexion, hip extension, and external rotation of the knee. The biceps femoris is the most frequently injured hamstring muscle, primarily due to its significant role in sprinting mechanics and eccentric force absorption. The semitendinosus, located medially, originates from the ischial tuberosity and inserts onto the pes anserinus of the medial tibia. This muscle is crucial in knee flexion, hip extension, and internal rotation of the knee. Its elongated tendon structure makes it particularly susceptible to tendinopathy especially in individuals with poor hamstring flexibility or excessive training loads. The semimembranosus, the deepest of the three hamstrings also originates from the ischial tuberosity but has a broader insertion at the posterior medial tibial condyle. It contributes significantly to knee stability by reinforcing the posterior knee capsule and reducing anterior tibial translation. This mechanism helps to protect against anterior cruciate ligament (ACL) injuries. The three muscles work in synergy to provide structural support, force generation, and controlled movement across the lower limb. Their coordinated function is essential for maintaining joint stability, neuromuscular efficiency, and optimal movement mechanics (Rodgers CD, 2023).

Biomechanical Function of the Hamstrings

The hamstrings fulfill several biomechanical functions based on movement requirements. Their principal function is knee flexion which is crucial for basic actions including walking, running, and kicking. During knee flexion, the biceps femoris externally rotates the tibia while the semitendinosus and semimembranosus medially rotate it which facilitates smooth joint articulation and mitigating excessive rotational stress at the knee. In addition to knee flexion, the hamstrings significantly contribute to hip extension, especially in actions necessitating propulsion and power generation. In collaboration with the gluteus maximus, they enable effective force transmission during the late stance phase of gait, promoting forward momentum and good stride mechanics. Their function in pelvic stability is crucial, since they regulate anterior pelvic tilt, alleviating stress on the lower back and sacroiliac joint. The hamstrings have a vital role in eccentric control during deceleration especially in high-velocity activities such as running. During sprinting, the hamstrings elongate under stress to regulate knee extension as the foot nears ground contact. This unconventional action is essential for mitigating the risk of ACL injury, since it counterbalances excessive anterior displacement of the tibia, which can impose excessive strain on the ligament(Ramos GA, 2017). Likewise, the hamstrings serve as shock absorbers upon landing, mitigating impact forces and averting knee hyperextension. Compromised hamstring flexibility or strength diminishes movement efficiency and frequently leads to compensatory patterns. Individuals with limited hamstring flexibility may encounter modified gait mechanics, heightened lumbar strain, and an increased susceptibility to lower limb injuries. This underscores the need to preserve hamstring flexibility and neuromuscular control to enhance optimal functional mobility and athletic performance(Opar DA, 2012).

Common Causes of Hamstring Tightness

Hamstring stiffness frequently arises from muscular imbalances, movement dysfunctions, and lifestyle influences. A predominant cause is prolonged sitting which maintains the hamstrings in a contracted state for protracted durations. Ultimately, this results in adaptive shortening, less elasticity, and a restricted range of motion, leading to stiffness and postural compensation. Muscle imbalances, especially quadriceps dominance, may result in pronounced hamstring tightness. Numerous athletes particularly in disciplines necessitating explosive power and sprinting frequently over utilise their quadriceps while inadequately engaging their posterior chain muscles. This imbalance exerts undue stress on the hamstrings which results in stiffness and a heightened risk of strains. Moreover, underdeveloped glutes compel the hamstrings to compensate during hip extension hence intensifying stiffness and dysfunction. A prevalent cause of hamstring tightness is inadequate rehabilitation and flexibility training. Individuals who perform high-intensity eccentric loading without sufficient mobility training encounter heightened muscular tension and microtrauma, resulting in gradual stiffness over time. Additionally, neurological variables such as sciatic nerve stress will lead to felt hamstring tightness, as defensive muscle guarding mechanisms restrict movement to avert further strain or injury. (LIYANAGE E, 2024).

Relevance to the Study: Why Understanding Hamstring Biomechanics Matters

This study examines the short-term impacts of two manual therapy techniques: Mulligan Bent Leg Raise (BLR) and Proprioceptive Neuromuscular Facilitation (PNF) Hold-Relax with Agonist Contraction (HR-AC) on enhancing hamstring flexibility and functional movement performance. Comprehending hamstring biomechanics is crucial for identifying the most effective strategy to restore optimal mobility, mitigate injury risk, and improve movement efficiency. A comprehensive grasp of the hamstring function in dynamic activities, eccentric control, and joint stabilization enables physiotherapists to customize rehabilitation programs efficiently. This study compares Mulligan BLR and PNF HR-AC to show the effects of manual therapy interventions on range of motion, neuromuscular activation, and movement efficiency, thereby informing best practices in physiotherapy and sports rehabilitation.

1.3 The Modern Epidemic: Hamstring Tightness in Sedentary and Active Populations

The Prevalence of Hamstring Tightness

Hamstring tightness has emerged as a significant musculoskeletal concern affecting both sedentary individuals and physically active populations. While it is often assumed that only athletes suffer from hamstring issues, research suggests that prolonged inactivity is equally detrimental to muscle flexibility. Sedentary individuals, particularly those who spend extended hours sitting at desks, in vehicles, or at home, frequently experience adaptive muscle shortening and postural imbalances. This leads to chronic tightness, decreased elasticity, and movement inefficiencies that contribute to long-term musculoskeletal discomfort. In contrast, athletes and highly active individuals develop hamstring tightness due to overuse, eccentric loading, and muscle imbalances, which result in increased muscle tone, reduced range of motion (ROM), and a heightened risk of injury. Whether due to inactivity or excessive mechanical stress, hamstring tightness compromises biomechanical efficiency, joint stability, and overall movement performance. Understanding how lifestyle and activity levels influence hamstring flexibility is essential for developing effective intervention strategies that restore muscle function and enhance movement efficiency(Jandre Reis FJ, 2015).

Hamstring Tightness in Sedentary Individuals

A sedentary lifestyle is one of the most common contributors to hamstring tightness in modern society. Millions of individuals spend prolonged hours in seated positions, either at work, in vehicles, or during leisure activities. This prolonged sitting keeps the hamstrings in a shortened state for extended periods, leading to a gradual loss of extensibility and neuromuscular deconditioning. Over time, the persistent lack of movement contributes to postural deviations, decreased flexibility, and functional limitations that impair mobility and increase the risk of chronic pain(Yadav R, 2020).

One of the most significant outcomes of extended sitting is the adaptive shortening of the hamstring muscles. When muscles are tightened for an extended period, structural changes occur that limit their ability to elongate efficiently. This is concerning for people who involve long periods of sitting labor as their hamstrings remain semi-contracted throughout the day. As a result, persistent tightness develops, reducing hip flexion, posterior chain mobility, and overall movement quality. Furthermore, prolonged inactivity causes neuromuscular deconditioning, resulting in diminished muscle flexibility and increased passive stiffness. (Spernoga SG, 2025).

Hamstring Tightness in Athletes and Physically Active Populations

Contrary to the assumption that physical activity prevents muscle tightness, athletes and highly active individuals are equally prone to hamstring dysfunction. While regular movement promotes muscle health, sports that involve rapid accelerations, sprinting, and high-impact landings place intense mechanical stress on the hamstrings, increasing the risk of chronic stiffness and overuse injuries. One of the most significant contributors to hamstring tightness in athletes is eccentric overload. Sports such as soccer, basketball, and track & field require explosive sprinting and sudden directional changes that place excessive strain on the hamstrings. These activities demand high levels of eccentric contraction, where the hamstrings lengthen under tension to decelerate movement. Over time, repeated eccentric loading causes microtrauma, which leads to increased muscle tone, reduced flexibility, and a greater likelihood of strain injuries. Muscle imbalances also play a crucial role in hamstring tightness among athletes. Many develop quadriceps dominance, where the anterior chain muscles including the quadriceps and hip flexors are overactive while the posterior chain comprising the hamstrings and glutes remains underdeveloped(Maniar N, 2021).

Postural Adaptations and Their Impact on Hamstring Flexibility

Both sedentary and athletic populations experience postural changes due to repetitive movement patterns, which significantly influence hamstring flexibility, and function. These postural adaptations lead to altered pelvic positioning, reduced joint mobility, and increased muscular tension, reinforcing hamstring tightness. In sedentary individuals, prolonged sitting frequently induces a posterior pelvic tilt which shortens the hamstrings and restricts hip mobility. Conversely, athletes with overactive hip flexors often develop an anterior pelvic tilt which places excessive strain on the hamstrings(López-Miñarro P, 2012).

The Role of Manual Therapy in Addressing Hamstring Tightness

Given the widespread prevalence of hamstring tightness across different populations, conventional static stretching alone is often insufficient in restoring optimal ROM and muscle function. Manual therapy techniques, such as Mulligan Bent Leg Raise (BLR) and PNF Hold-Relax (HR-AC), offer targeted interventions that enhance neuromuscular activation, improve muscle elasticity, and facilitate immediate gains in flexibility.

1.4 Limitations in Daily Functional Activities

Introduction: The Role of Hamstring Flexibility in Daily Life

Hamstring flexibility is a critical determinant of mobility and movement efficiency, playing an essential role in activities such as walking, standing, bending, and reaching. While often linked to athletic performance, the importance of hamstring flexibility extends far beyond sports, influencing everyday functional movements across various age groups and activity levels. The hamstring muscles work in coordination with the hip extensors and knee flexors to allow smooth, controlled movement. When hamstring extensibility is compromised, movement restrictions arise leading to postural compensations, inefficient biomechanics, chronic discomfort, and increased susceptibility to musculoskeletal injuries. Restricted hamstring flexibility results in compensatory movement patterns, forcing other muscle groups and joints to absorb excessive strain. Over time, this compensation alters neuromuscular control, increases muscular imbalances, and predisposes individuals to chronic pain syndromes that hinder functional independence. In individuals engaged in physically demanding jobs or recreational activities, tight hamstrings reduce movement efficiency increasing the likelihood of strain-related injuries. Conversely, those with sedentary lifestyles experience progressive stiffness and mobility deficits, further contributing to postural misalignment and movement dysfunctions. Addressing hamstring tightness through targeted interventions is essential for maintaining optimal musculoskeletal health, preventing mobility-related disorders, and enhancing the overall quality of life(Wan X, 2020).

Impaired Mobility and Reduced Range of Motion (ROM)

One of the most immediate and functionally limiting consequences of hamstring tightness is a reduction in active and passive ROM, particularly affecting knee extension and hip flexion.

These limitations significantly impair activities that require dynamic movement and unrestricted joint mobility, affecting individuals in both active and sedentary populations. For instance, daily tasks such as bending to tie shoelaces, lifting objects, or reaching for items on a lower shelf demand sufficient hamstring extensibility. Individuals with tight hamstrings often compensate by excessively rounding their lower back, increasing strain on the lumbar spine. This postural misalignment amplifies pressure on the intervertebral discs, potentially leading to lower back discomfort, spinal rigidity, and an increased risk of lumbar dysfunctions such as disc herniation. Hamstring tightness also affects sitting and standing postures, particularly in individuals who spend prolonged periods in static positions. When seated, tight hamstrings pull the pelvis into a posterior tilt, altering natural spinal alignment and shifting weight distribution in the lower back and sacral region. This leads to lumbar pressure buildup, increasing the risk of chronic pain, postural imbalances, and muscular fatigue. Over time, restricted hamstring flexibility leads to movement inefficiencies, forcing the body to adopt compensatory kinematic patterns that further contribute to discomfort and an increased risk of musculoskeletal injuries (Konrad et al., 2024).

Postural Compensations and Their Impact on Daily Life

When hamstring flexibility is compromised, the body naturally adopts postural compensations to maintain movement efficiency. However, these compensatory patterns often lead to long-term musculoskeletal dysfunctions, increasing the risk of chronic pain, reduced movement efficiency, and susceptibility to injury. One of the most common postural adaptations seen in individuals with tight hamstrings is a posterior pelvic tilt, where the pelvis is pulled downward due to the shortened hamstring length. This flattening of the natural lumbar curve negatively impacts spinal alignment and core stability, limiting the spine's ability to absorb shock and distribute mechanical loads effectively. Over time, this misalignment increases tension in the lower back, predisposing individuals to disc degeneration, sciatic nerve compression, and chronic lumbar stiffness. In dynamic movements, individuals with restricted hamstring mobility compensate by overactivating adjacent muscle groups, leading to inefficient movement mechanics. For example, in walking and running, reduced hamstring extensibility forces the hip flexors to become overactive, altering stride length and increasing ground reaction forces on the knees and ankles. These maladaptive movement patterns reduce movement efficiency, increase energy expenditure, and predispose individuals to lower-limb overuse injuries(Encarnación-Martínez A, 2023).

Effects on Workplace Ergonomics and Productivity

Hamstring tightness is a major contributing factor to workplace inefficiency, ergonomic discomfort, and musculoskeletal fatigue, particularly in occupations that involve prolonged sitting, repetitive movements, or physically demanding tasks. For office workers and professionals who remain seated for extended durations, hamstring shortening becomes a persistent issue due to the continuous maintenance of a contracted muscle position. This not only restricts hip mobility but also induces lumbar stiffness, sacral pressure buildup, and spinal discomfort, ultimately leading to postural fatigue, loss of concentration, and reduced productivity. In contrast, physically active workers, such as laborers, factory workers, and construction professionals, rely heavily on lower-limb mobility and flexibility to perform lifting, squatting, and dynamic postural transitions. Hamstring tightness in these individuals limits movement efficiency, increasing the risk of improper lifting mechanics, lumbar strain, and work-related musculoskeletal disorders (WMSDs). Given these occupational implications, corrective flexibility training and manual therapy interventions are crucial for improving ergonomic performance and minimizing the risk of work-related injuries (Gou Y, 2024)

Impact on Aging and Fall Risk in Older Adults

In aging populations, hamstring flexibility directly influences mobility, stability, and fall risk. As individuals age, muscle elasticity naturally declines, reducing the capacity for efficient movement and postural adjustments. Hamstring tightness in older adults leads to restricted hip and knee mobility, impairing their ability to maintain proper postural alignment and balance. A lack of lower-limb flexibility negatively affects gait mechanics, often resulting in shorter stride lengths, increased reliance on visual feedback for movement navigation, and an overall decline in functional independence. Additionally, older individuals with compromised hamstring extensibility experience reduced proprioceptive feedback, making them more prone to falls and sudden balance disturbances. Diminished reaction times and postural compensations such as excessive forward trunk lean during ambulation further elevate the risk of falls and lower extremity injuries. As falls remain a leading cause of morbidity in aging populations, maintaining hamstring flexibility through targeted interventions is essential for prolonging mobility and functional autonomy(Haab T, 2017).

1.5 Athletic Performance and Injury Risks

The Role of Hamstring Flexibility in Athletic Performance

Hamstring flexibility is a cornerstone of athletic performance, playing a crucial role in enabling explosive movements, controlling joint mechanics, and minimizing the risk of injury. In nearly all sports, from sprinting and jumping to cutting, pivoting, and rapid changes of direction, the hamstrings act as key functional contributors to both propulsive and stabilizing phases of motion. Their role as biarticular muscles, spanning both the hip and knee joints, gives them a dual function in coordinating complex limb movements. Optimal hamstring extensibility allows for full hip extension and knee flexion, contributing to efficient force transmission, stride length, and shock absorption all essential elements of high-level performance. When hamstring flexibility is reduced, the resulting biomechanical limitations can severely impair athletic capacity. A tight hamstring complex not only restricts hip range but also reduces the ability of the knee to move dynamically and efficiently during explosive movements. This compromises muscle synergy, disrupts force sequencing, and impairs overall neuromuscular control, leading to suboptimal performance and a significantly elevated injury risk. Sports that involve repeated eccentric loading such as sprinting, jumping, and lunging are particularly affected by these limitations as eccentric control requires sufficient muscle length and elasticity to safely absorb and redirect high mechanical forces(Wan X, 2017).

Impaired Sprinting and Acceleration Mechanics

In high-intensity sports such as football, rugby, track and field, and basketball, sprinting and acceleration mechanics are central to an athlete's competitive edge. These dynamic movements require a high degree of lower limb coordination, optimal hip mobility, and timed eccentric and concentric muscle activity, with the hamstrings playing a pivotal role in these phases. One of the most significant impacts of hamstring tightness is on stride mechanics. Stride length, a major determinant of sprint speed, is highly dependent on the ability of the hip to extend through its full range. When hamstrings are tight, hip extension is restricted, and athletes are forced to take shorter, quicker steps to maintain speed. This increases step frequency, elevates energy expenditure, and reduces mechanical efficiency, ultimately resulting in slower sprint times and premature fatigue. The hamstrings also serve a crucial function during the late swing phase of sprinting, where they contract eccentrically to decelerate the forward momentum of the tibia and stabilize the knee joint before foot contact. If the hamstring is too tight, this phase is compromised—deceleration occurs too late or inefficiently, resulting in increased muscle strain and mechanical overload, particularly at the myotendinous junction, a common site for hamstring tears. Moreover, explosive acceleration, which requires a powerful hip extension, becomes significantly impaired when hamstring flexibility is limited. Athletes are unable to drive their hips through a full range, leading to a compromised force production chain, reducing ground reaction force generation and decreasing acceleration capacity(Prince C, 2021).

Increased Risk of Hamstring Strains and Muscle Injuries

Hamstring injuries rank among the most common and recurrent injuries in sports, especially in activities that include sprinting, sudden halting, and directional changes. A primary risk factor for hamstring strain injuries is insufficient flexibility coupled with inadequate eccentric control. During high-velocity running, the muscles experience fast eccentric contractions, particularly in the terminal swing phase, when they extend while contracting to decelerate the leg. When flexibility is constrained, the muscle is positioned in a more precarious state, functioning at its full length with inadequate compliance to accommodate the mechanical load(Gaku Tokutake, 2018). This increases tensile stress within the muscle fibers, predisposing them to microtrauma and partial or full-thickness tears. Additionally, tight hamstrings compromise neuromuscular efficiency, leading to delayed activation and reduced stabilization capacity at the hip and knee joints. This diminished responsiveness increases the risk of uncontrolled movement, especially in fatigue states where motor control declines. Compensatory reliance on synergist muscles such as the quadriceps and lumbar extensors. This introduces biomechanical asymmetry, overloads non-target tissues, and increases the risk of secondary injuries to the spine or anterior knee structures(Buckthorpe M, 2018).

The Link Between Hamstring Tightness and ACL Injuries

The hamstrings function as dynamic stabilizers of the knee joint by counteracting anterior tibial translation, a movement that may jeopardize the integrity of the anterior cruciate ligament (ACL) if performed excessively. Restricted hamstring flexibility hinders the muscle's ability to activate and contract efficiently, thereby diminishing its protective function during high-risk activities such as jumping, landing, and pivoting. ACL injuries frequently occur in sports that demand rapid deceleration and directional changes, including soccer, basketball, and skiing. Limited hamstring flexibility alters landing mechanics, often resulting in stiffer landings, reduced hip flexion, and increased knee valgus—all recognized risk factors for non-contact ACL injury. Without adequate flexibility, athletes are less able to absorb landing forces effectively, transferring mechanical stress directly to ligament structures. In addition, hamstring tightness may impair proprioceptive feedback and joint awareness, leading athletes to misjudge limb position and increasing the likelihood of poor alignment and elevated ACL strain. Evidence indicates that flexibility-focused interventions such as the Mulligan Bent Leg Raise and kinetic chain activation not only improve hamstring extensibility but also enhance neuromuscular control of the knee, thereby supporting safer landing strategies and reducing ACL injury risk (Sos Tirado et al., 2024).

The Role of Hamstring Flexibility in Injury Recovery

Hamstring flexibility is not only a protective factor but also a critical component of post-injury rehabilitation. After injuries such as hamstring strains, ACL reconstruction, or lumbar spine dysfunction, restoring hamstring extensibility is essential for re-establishing normal movement patterns, reducing recurrence risk, and promoting long-term tissue health. Following a hamstring strain, the development of fibrotic scar tissue at the injury site reduces elasticity and creates focal areas of stiffness. Without targeted flexibility interventions, this stiffness can become chronic, predisposing the athlete to re-injury during high-velocity or high-load movements. Manual therapy techniques, including deep tissue release and proprioceptive stretching, help break down adhesions, remodel collagen fibers, and restore tissue compliance(Sugiura Y, 2017). Moreover, after ACL reconstruction or knee trauma, hamstring flexibility becomes a limiting factor in restoring gait symmetry, balance, and sports-specific skills. Patients with post-surgical tightness often adopt compensatory movement strategies that overload the contralateral limb or trunk, leading to a cascade of mechanical imbalances. Integrating hamstring stretching into rehabilitation programs enhances neuromuscular re-education, improves dynamic control, and ensures efficient return-to-play outcomes.

The Need for Manual Therapy Interventions in Athletes

Given the multifaceted effects of hamstring tightness on performance restrictions, injury risk, and delayed recovery, focused manual therapy interventions are essential for athletes of all levels. Techniques like Mulligan Bent Leg Raise (BLR) and PNF Hold-Relax with Agonist Contraction (HR-AC) have gained popularity because they actively engage the neuromuscular system and restore flexibility more effectively than static or passive stretching. Mulligan BLR combines joint mobilization with active engagement to correct movement errors while improving hip and hamstring mobility. It is particularly effective for individuals with joint-related flexibility deficits and can be incorporated into warm-up and recovery regimens to enhance athletic performance. PNF HR-AC, by contrast, utilizes isometric contractions followed by relaxation and stretching to achieve deeper muscle elongation and substantial ROM improvements. Both methods significantly improve hamstring extensibility, and recent evidence confirms that BLR produces clinically meaningful short-term gains in range of motion and functional mobility. Furthermore, comparative findings show that BLR is equally effective as the Kinetic Chain Activation Technique in enhancing hamstring length and movement efficiency, reinforcing its value as a reliable intervention across athletic and rehabilitation settings (Santosh C M, 2025).

1.6 The Mulligan Bent Leg Raise (BLR) Technique

Manual Therapy and the Needs for Mulligan Mobilization

Manual therapy has long been a cornerstone in the physiotherapeutic management of musculoskeletal dysfunctions. Its role in addressing joint restrictions, muscular tightness, and soft tissue impairments is well-documented, particularly in populations experiencing chronic stiffness, limited range of motion (ROM), and movement inefficiencies. Among the wide array of manual therapy approaches, the Mulligan Concept, developed by New Zealand physiotherapist Brian Mulligan, has gained significant attention for its unique emphasis on Mobilization with Movement (MWM). This technique integrates passive joint mobilization with active patient participation to promote functional improvements without inducing pain or resistance. The Mulligan Bent Leg Raise (BLR) technique is a specialized application of the MWM concept, designed specifically to target hamstring flexibility, neuromuscular control, and lower limb joint kinematics. Unlike conventional static stretching, which primarily seeks to elongate the muscle-tendon unit through passive means, Mulligan BLR incorporates a joint-based mobilization strategy combined with isometric muscular contraction. This creates a multimodal therapeutic input, simultaneously influencing joint arthrokinematics, muscle extensibility, and sensorimotor control. Given the widespread presence of hamstring tightness in both sedentary and athletic populations, the Mulligan BLR offers a non-invasive, functional, and evidence-informed alternative for clinicians aiming to improve hamstring ROM, optimize hip and knee mechanics, and prevent strain-related injuries. The growing interest in this technique stems from its clinical efficiency, patient tolerance, and long-term functional benefits across a wide range of movement disorders(Stathopoulos N, 2019).

Biomechanical Principles and Execution of the Mulligan BLR Technique

At its core, the Mulligan BLR technique is built on the foundation of Mobilization with Movement (MWM), a principle that emphasizes simultaneous passive joint mobilization and active patient engagement. This differs fundamentally from static stretching approaches by introducing movement variability, joint correction, and neuromuscular control into a single intervention. The goal is to normalize joint biomechanics, enhance proprioceptive signaling, and improve muscular extensibility in a functional, movement-specific context.

Step-by-Step Execution of the Mulligan BLR:

1. Patient Positioning:

The patient lies in a supine position with the target leg flexed at both the hip and knee. Proper alignment of the pelvis and lumbar spine is ensured to minimize compensatory trunk movements that could confound the effectiveness of the technique. Positioning is crucial, as it sets the foundation for targeted joint mobilization and safe muscle activation.

2. Active Patient Engagement:

Next, the patient is instructed to gently push their leg against the therapist's shoulder in an isometric contraction, typically held for around 8 seconds. This contraction activates the hamstrings without producing joint movement. After the contraction, a relaxation phase is performed during which the therapist gently increases hip flexion thereby stretching the hamstrings. This combination of isometric loading followed by passive elongation helps facilitate deeper flexibility gains through autogenic inhibition.

3. Repetition and Progression:

The entire sequence is repeated approximately 10 times, each time aiming to progressively increase the angle of hip flexion. Importantly, the therapist continues to apply the joint glide throughout each repetition, ensuring that joint alignment and mobility are continuously optimized. This repetition protocol ensures gradual tissue adaptation, minimizing strain and enhancing long-term neuromuscular and connective tissue remodeling.

Mechanisms of Action: How the Mulligan BLR Improves Flexibility

The clinical efficacy of the Mulligan BLR is underpinned by a combination of neuromuscular, biomechanical, and sensorimotor mechanisms. These mechanisms work synergistically to produce rapid and measurable gains in flexibility, while also contributing to longer-term improvements in movement efficiency and control.

Neural Desensitization and Reduction of Muscle Spasms

Hamstring tightness often involves not only mechanical resistance but also neural sensitivity and protective muscle guarding, particularly in individuals with a history of injury. The Mulligan BLR technique has been shown to reduce alpha-motor neuron excitability, thereby lowering muscle tone and spasm activity. By modulating the central and peripheral nervous systems, the technique allows the muscle to elongate without triggering a stretch reflex, facilitating greater ROM without discomfort(Adnan M, 2021).

Enhanced Joint Glide and Hip-Pelvis Mechanics

Joint mobilization within the BLR technique addresses arthrokinematic restrictions, which often contribute to perceived muscular tightness. By mobilizing the hip joint, therapists improve capsular elasticity and joint congruency, which in turn allows for more effective hamstring elongation. Additionally, improved pelvic mobility supports a more functional lumbopelvic rhythm during flexion and extension tasks.

Facilitated Proprioceptive Feedback and Motor Control

Incorporating active isometric contractions into the BLR sequence enhances proprioceptive feedback loops between the hamstrings and the central nervous system. This reeducation of neuromuscular pathways improves muscle coordination, joint positioning, and reflexive activation, ultimately contributing to a reduction in tightness recurrence. The proprioceptive enhancement also plays a key role in injury prevention, as it improves an athlete's ability to respond to rapid movement demands(P. M, 2023).

Autogenic Inhibition via Golgi Tendon Organ Activation

The isometric contraction phase of the Mulligan BLR stimulates the Golgi Tendon Organs (GTOs) within the hamstring musculature. Activation of the GTOs induces autogenic inhibition, a reflex that results in the relaxation of the contracted muscle, thereby allowing it to be passively stretched further and more comfortably. This reflex mechanism is central to the increased flexibility gains observed following Mulligan BLR interventions(Sita A, 2021).

Clinical Applications of Mulligan BLR in Hamstring Rehabilitation

The Mulligan BLR technique is widely utilized across clinical, athletic, and rehabilitative settings, given its applicability in managing both acute and chronic flexibility impairments. Its versatility lies in its non-invasive nature, rapid effectiveness, and patient-centered execution.

Chronic Hamstring Tightness

In both sedentary and athletic individuals, persistent hamstring tightness can alter normal lumbopelvic mechanics, reduce functional mobility, and increase susceptibility to strain injuries.

The Mulligan BLR offers a gentle yet targeted method for increasing ROM and reducing muscle resistance. It is particularly effective for individuals who do not tolerate traditional static or ballistic stretching due to discomfort or low compliance (Hall T, 2006). Recent systematic reviews reinforce these observations: Hussein et al. (2025) confirmed BLR's effectiveness in improving hamstring flexibility and functional outcomes, while ElMeligie et al. (2025) demonstrated that mobilization-with-movement interventions also improve ROM and neuromuscular control in related musculoskeletal conditions.

Post-Injury Rehabilitation (e.g., Hamstring Strains, ACL Recovery)

After a hamstring strain or ACL reconstruction, patients often develop protective stiffness and compensatory movement patterns. The Mulligan BLR serves as a mid-phase rehabilitative technique, helping restore ROM while reintroducing neuromuscular control in a controlled manner. It also reduces the risk of recurring injury by improving tissue extensibility and alignment without inducing aggressive strain(Sivasubramanian K, 2022).

Athletic Performance Enhancement

In elite sports, performance hinges on explosive movements, sprinting mechanics, and neuromuscular reactivity. The Mulligan BLR technique is used to improve stride length, hip extension efficiency, and acceleration capacity. Incorporating the technique into warm-ups and recovery sessions helps maintain functional mobility and reduce the cumulative risk of injury in high-volume athletes.

Management of Lower Back Pain and Postural Dysfunction

Tight hamstrings often contribute to posterior pelvic tilt and lumbar spine flattening, leading to lower back pain and poor postural mechanics. The Mulligan BLR's dual effect on joint mobility and muscle length helps correct these imbalances, facilitating a neutral spine position and improved trunk-pelvis coordination(Adnan M, 2022).

Why Compare Mulligan BLR with PNF Hold-Relax?

Despite its growing popularity and clinical success, the Mulligan BLR technique has not been extensively compared with other evidence-based interventions, particularly PNF Hold-Relax with Agonist Contraction. PNF is known for its ability to induce rapid neuromuscular relaxation and muscle elongation through isometric contraction and post-contraction stretching. Comparing the Mulligan Bent Leg Raise (BLR) technique and the Proprioceptive Neuromuscular Facilitation (PNF) Hold-Relax method enables clinicians and researchers to critically evaluate the relative efficacy of each approach. This comparison facilitates the identification of which technique is more effective in producing immediate improvements in the hamstring range of motion. It also allows for an examination of whether Mulligan BLR provides superior outcomes in terms of neuromuscular coordination and proprioceptive enhancement when compared to PNF. Furthermore, evaluating both interventions helps determine how patients perceive each method in terms of comfort, tolerance, and the level of control they experience during application. Finally, this analysis contributes to understanding the differential long-term effects of each technique, particularly with regard to injury recurrence rates and the normalization of functional movement patterns.

1.7 The Proprioceptive Neuromuscular Facilitation (PNF) Hold-Relax with Agonist Contraction (HR-AC) Technique

The Role of PNF in Enhancing Flexibility

Proprioceptive Neuromuscular Facilitation is a well-established manual therapy technique designed to enhance flexibility, muscle strength, and neuromuscular coordination. Originally developed in the mid-20th century for neurological rehabilitation, PNF has since been widely adopted in sports science, physiotherapy, and rehabilitation medicine due to its effectiveness in increasing the range of motion and improving functional movement patterns. Among the various PNF techniques, the Hold-Relax with Agonist Contraction method is recognized as one of the most effective interventions for improving hamstring flexibility and muscle performance. This technique is unique because it combines passive stretching, isometric contraction, and active engagement of the antagonist muscle group, allowing for neuromuscular adaptation and functional mobility enhancement. By utilizing autogenic and reciprocal inhibition mechanisms, PNF HR-AC optimizes muscle relaxation, stretch tolerance, and movement efficiency, making it particularly useful for athletes, rehabilitation patients, and individuals with chronic muscle tightness. Given the importance of hamstring flexibility in athletic performance, injury prevention, and postural alignment, the PNF HR-AC technique provides a clinically validated approach to optimizing mobility. This section explores the biomechanical principles, physiological mechanisms, and clinical applications of PNF HR-AC, emphasizing its role in hamstring rehabilitation and performance enhancement(Rahul Krishnan Kutty, 2023).

Biomechanical Principles and Execution of the PNF HR-AC Technique

The PNF HR-AC technique is based on two key neuromuscular principles. The first is autogenic inhibition, where a muscle's Golgi Tendon Organs (GTOs) detect tension during an isometric contraction, leading to a reflexive reduction in muscle tone that allows the muscle to relax and perform further stretch. The second key component is reciprocal inhibition, a process in which the activation of the agonist muscle (quadriceps in this case) signals the nervous system to inhibit the antagonist muscle (hamstrings), reducing resistance and facilitating greater ROM improvements. These physiological responses enable immediate and progressive gains in muscle flexibility, making PNF HR-AC particularly effective for both static and dynamic movement applications. To properly execute the PNF HR-AC technique, the patient is positioned on their side with their unaffected leg extended and anchored over the side of the treatment table for additional stabilization. The therapist then lifts the affected leg into hip flexion with the knee extended, applying a gentle passive stretch to the hamstrings. Once the patient reaches a mild stretch, the isometric hold phase begins. During this phase, the patient is instructed to push their leg downward against the therapist's resistance for 8 seconds, a duration supported by recent stretching protocols as sufficient to activate autogenic inhibition. This isometric contraction stimulates the GTOs, initiating autogenic inhibition, which reduces muscle tension and increases stretch tolerance ('Comparison Between SLR and BLR Stretching Techniques,' 2024).

Following the isometric contraction, the patient enters the relaxation phase, during which they completely release any effort. This allows the therapist to passively move the leg further into hip flexion, increasing the stretch depth. This phase takes advantage of temporary muscle relaxation, allowing for greater elongation without excessive discomfort. Immediately after, the agonist contraction phase begins, in which the patient actively contracts the quadriceps to further lift the leg into hip flexion. This action engages reciprocal inhibition, causing additional relaxation in the hamstrings and allowing for deeper elongation. The entire sequence is repeated three to five times per session, with each repetition gradually increasing ROM. The combination of isometric contraction, passive stretching, and active movement makes PNF HR-AC one of the most effective interventions for immediate and long-term flexibility gains(Pourahmadi M, 2020).

Mechanisms of Action: How PNF HR-AC Improves Flexibility

The effectiveness of the PNF HR-AC technique can be connected with several key neuromuscular and biomechanical mechanisms that facilitate muscle relaxation and elongation. One of the primary mechanisms is the inhibition of the stretch reflex. Normally, the muscle spindle reflex resists rapid muscle elongation by triggering a protective contraction. However, in PNF stretching, this reflex is temporarily suppressed during the isometric contraction and relaxation phases which allows the hamstring muscle to stretch beyond its usual limits without triggering involuntary resistance. Another contributing factor is increased stretch tolerance, which occurs as repeated PNF stretching sessions train the nervous system to accept greater muscle elongation with reduced discomfort. This adaptation is particularly beneficial for athletes and individuals recovering from musculoskeletal injuries, as it enables greater functional ROM. Additionally, PNF HR-AC improves neuromuscular coordination by activating the agonist muscle (quadriceps), which reduces compensatory movement patterns commonly observed in individuals with chronic hamstring tightness or movement restrictions. Unlike passive stretching, which simply elongates the muscle, PNF HR-AC also strengthens end-range control, reinforcing active muscle engagement and improving eccentric control in lengthened positions. This increased control is crucial for sports performance and rehabilitation settings, where functional flexibility is required for explosive movements and injury prevention(Youdas JW, 2010).

Clinical Applications of PNF HR-AC in Hamstring Rehabilitation

The PNF HR-AC approach is extensively employed in physiotherapy, sports medicine and rehabilitation due to its efficacy in swiftly enhancing flexibility, and reinstating functional movement patterns. A prevalent application is in the rehabilitation of hamstring strains, where it facilitates the regulated elongation of muscle fibers, hence diminishing the chance of re-injury and enhancing movement efficiency. It is also commonly used in post-surgical knee and hip rehabilitation, particularly following ACL reconstruction or total knee replacement, as it enhances ROM and strength balance between the hamstrings and quadriceps. In sports performance enhancement, PNF HR-AC is used to optimize sprint acceleration and kicking mechanics, improving dynamic flexibility and power output in athletes who require rapid deceleration and directional changes. Additionally, the technique is effective in managing chronic lower back pain, as tight hamstrings contribute to posterior pelvic tilt and lumbar dysfunction. By improving lumbar-pelvic mobility, PNF HR-AC reduces strain on the lower back and improves postural alignment(de Sire A, 2024).

Comparing PNF HR-AC with Mulligan BLR

Although PNF HR-AC is a well-documented intervention, research directly comparing its effectiveness with the Mulligan Bent Leg Raise (BLR) technique remains limited. Both techniques aim to enhance hamstring mobility, but they differ in mechanisms and therapeutic approaches. The PNF HR-AC technique utilizes neuromuscular inhibition mechanisms, whereas the Mulligan BLR technique focuses on joint mobilization and positional correction. Additionally, PNF HR-AC actively engages the antagonist muscle, while Mulligan BLR applies passive and active-assisted mobilization. Due to variations in patient comfort and responses, additional study is necessary to discover the most effective approach for diverse patient populations. This study will offer essential insights into the most effective intervention for enhancing hamstring flexibility and functional mobility by directly comparing these two strategies.

1.0 Research Objectives

This study aims to compare two manual therapy techniques, the Mulligan Bent Leg Raise (BLR) and Proprioceptive Neuromuscular Facilitation (PNF) Hold-Relax with Agonist Contraction, focusing on their effectiveness on hamstring flexibility, muscle performance, patient comfort, and preference. These objectives will generate evidence to guide physiotherapists in selecting effective, patient-centered interventions.

1.Assess Direct Effect on Hamstring range of motion:

The goal is to determine the way each technique impacts hamstring range of motion, which is vital for effective movement and prevention of injuries. The study examines ROM before and after the intervention to find out which approach provides a significant rise in flexibility. The findings will give physiotherapists important new information when working with patients who have limited movement and tight hamstrings.

2.**Assess the effectiveness of the outcomes of muscle performance** Muscles need to be stabilized and strengthened for functional strength, particularly peak torque. This goal will evaluate each intervention's direct impact on muscle function. The results will help therapists determine the most efficient method to improve muscle strength and flexibility, which is crucial for both recovery and performance in sports.

3.**Identify Relevant Clinical Decision-Making Uses: This goal looks at each** technique's wider clinical applicability in addition to its physical outcomes. Physiotherapists can make evidence-based decisions for a range of patient populations, particularly those who need rapid flexibility gains, by using information about muscle function, range of motion and flexibility.

Problem statement:

1.**Lack of Comparative Analysis of Manual Therapy Techniques** Current rehabilitation practices for addressing hamstring flexibility and muscle performance often rely on established manual therapy techniques such as Mulligan Bent Leg Raise (BLR) and Proprioceptive Neuromuscular Facilitation (PNF) Hold-Relax with Agonist Contraction. However, the relative effectiveness of these two methods in improving hamstring range of motion and muscle performance remains underexplored. The lack of comparative analysis creates a significant gap in evidence-based physiotherapy which limits the ability of therapists to tailor interventions that are suitable for each individual.

2.**Insufficient Exploration of Mechanistic Differences** Although both Mulligan BLR and PNF Hold-Relax techniques are widely used, the underlying mechanisms by which they influence hamstring flexibility and muscle performance are not fully understood. Exploring how these techniques interact with neuromuscular and biomechanical pathways helps to provide deeper insights into their efficacy. This highlights the need for research focusing on the physiological and biomechanical processes activated by these interventions to provide clear insight into clinical practice.

Hypotheses

- **H0 (Null Hypothesis)**: There will be no significant difference in the immediate effects of the Mulligan BLR and PNF Hold-Relax with Agonist Contraction techniques on hamstring ROM, muscle performance, patient comfort, and technique preference.
- **H1 (Alternative Hypotheses)**: The Mulligan BLR technique will result in a significant increase in hamstring ROM compared to the PNF Hold-Relax with Agonist with Agonist Contraction technique.

Research question

What is the comparative efficacy of the Mulligan Bent Leg Raise technique versus the PNF Hold-Relax exercise in enhancing hamstring range of motion and muscle function in young people with restricted hamstring flexibility?

Objectives of research

Primary: To compare the efficacy of the Mulligan Bent Leg Raise technique and PNF Hold-Relax exercise in improving hamstring range of motion and muscle performance in young adults with limited hamstring flexibility.

Secondary: To investigate the specific contributions of the Mulligan Bent Leg Raise technique and PNF Hold-Relax exercise on clinically relevant outcomes, including hamstring range of motion measured using a goniometer in active knee extension and muscle performance assessed using a handheld dynamometer, in young adults with limited hamstring flexibility.

CHAPTER 2

Methodology

2.1Introduction

The research methodology is a randomized controlled trial. The research will be carried out at the Caring Bone Care Physiotherapy Center. The completion of this investigation is anticipated within 3 months. The overall sample size comprises 64 individuals, with 32 people allocated to each group. The sample size is determined with G*power 3.1.9.7. The convenient sampling approach will be employed. Participants must complete three visits. All participants will undergo baseline evaluations, encompassing hamstring range of motion examined with a goniometer and muscle performance recorded with a handheld dynamometer. Inclusion criteria encompass persons aged 18 to 35 years, regardless of gender, who exhibit restricted hamstring flexibility and are willing to participate. Outcome measures, including hamstring range of motion during active knee extension and muscle function, will be evaluated at baseline and upon completion of the 6-week intervention. Exclusion criteria encompass people with acute hamstring injuries occurring within the past 6 weeks, a history of lower extremity surgery, or any neurological or musculoskeletal disorders that impair lower limb function. This research will be a randomized controlled trial (RCT) comprising two intervention groups, each assigned one of the two approaches. Participants will be randomly allocated to either the Mulligan Bent Leg Raise (BLR) group or the PNF Hold-Relax group. Every participant is required to attend three sessions. Measurements of Active Knee Extension (utilizing a goniometer) and muscular performance (employing a hand-held dynamometer) will be conducted immediately before and after the intervention during each visit.

2.2 Sample Population

The study will involve 64 young adult participants aged 18-35 years, each with limited hamstring flexibility but no significant musculoskeletal or neurological conditions. This age group was chosen for its general physical health and adaptability to flexibility interventions, allowing for a clear assessment of technique effects.

2.3 Criteria

Criteria for Inclusion:

- **Participants:** must be between the ages of 18 and 35.
- **Baseline Flexibility:** People who, according to an Active Knee Extension Test, Knee remains >20° when flexed is consider hamstring tightness
- **Consent:** Individuals who have given their written, informed consent to take part in the research.
- **Availability:** People who are accessible throughout the study period.

Criteria for Exclusion:

- **Medical Conditions:** People with a history of lower limb neurological disorders, musculoskeletal injuries, or surgeries.
- **Prior Treatment:** People who, during the previous three months, received any kind of physiotherapy or lower limb muscle interventions.
- **Medications**: Participants taking medications that affect muscle function or pain perception, such as muscle relaxants or opioids.
- **Pregnancy**: Pregnant individuals due to potential risks and altered body mechanics affecting flexibility and muscle performance.

2.4 Sample Size Calculation

The required sample size of 64 participants (32 per group) was determined using G*Power 3.1 software, assuming an effect size of 0.8, a power of 80% ($\beta = 0.20$), and a significance level of $\alpha = 0.05$. A 10% dropout rate was factored into the final sample size estimation to account for participant attrition.

2.5 Recruitment Procedure

Participant recruitment will take place at Caring Bone Care Physiotherapy Center, where individuals seeking treatment or general musculoskeletal screening will be approached regarding their potential eligibility for the study. To ensure a normally distributed sample, participants will be recruited using a stratified sampling approach, dividing them into age subgroups (18–22, 23–26, 27–30 years) and gender subgroups (male and female) to achieve a balanced representation across different demographic groups. Potential participants will undergo an initial screening assessment conducted by licensed physiotherapists at the center, during which hamstring flexibility will be measured using the Active Knee Extension Test (AKET). In accordance with AKET criteria, an angle of 20° or more will be classified as hamstring tightness. Individuals who match the eligibility criteria will obtain a comprehensive study information sheet detailing goals, procedures, risks, and benefits of participation. Before enrolment, each participant will receive a written informed consent form which they must examine and sign before advancing with the study. Participants will be apprised of their entitlement to withdraw at any moment without consequences. To uphold a randomized distribution, a goal of about equal representation from each subgroup will be established, ensuring that the sample adheres to a normal distribution within the specified population range.

2.6 Randomization and Blinding

A computer-generated randomization sequence will be used to allocate participants into one of two intervention groups:

1. Mulligan Bent Leg Raise (BLR) Group (n=32)
2. PNF Hold-Relax (HR) Group (n=32)

This study employed a single-blinded design, wherein the outcome assessor was blinded to group allocation throughout the data collection and post-intervention measurement phases. This blinding strategy was strategically implemented to reduce the risk of observer bias, particularly during the assessment of subjective or semi-objective outcome measures such as range of motion and muscle strength. By ensuring that the assessor did not possess prior knowledge of which intervention: Mulligan Bent Leg Raise (BLR) or Proprioceptive Neuromuscular Facilitation (PNF) Hold-Relax of each participant received, the potential for influencing measurement techniques or expectations was significantly reduced. This approach strengthens the neutrality and objectivity of outcome evaluations, thereby enhancing the credibility of the observed effects.

Although full double-blinding was not feasible due to the hands-on nature of both interventions, where participants and therapists were necessarily aware of the technique being administered, care was taken to standardize the interaction and instructions given by the therapists to minimize performance bias. Both groups received interventions in identical clinical settings, using similar equipment and treatment durations, thereby controlling for environmental and procedural confounding variables. Furthermore, therapists were instructed to maintain a neutral tone and encouragement levels during both Mulligan and PNF sessions to avoid introducing subconscious reinforcement or preferential treatment that might influence patient effort or perception. To further mitigate bias, the random allocation sequence was concealed using sealed, opaque envelopes until the point of assignment, reducing the possibility of selection bias during the recruitment and grouping phases. The study also documented complete adherence and zero dropout rates, which eliminates the threat of attrition bias, a common concern in interventional trials where differential loss to follow-up can distort findings.

2.7 Intervention Protocol

Each intervention session will last for 30 minutes and will be conducted two times per week for a total of three weeks. The interventions will be performed by a licensed physiotherapist with clinical experience in musculoskeletal rehabilitation. Each technique will follow a standardized protocol to maintain consistency across sessions.

2.8 Expected Outcomes

The study is expected to yield immediate data on the effectiveness, comfort, and participant preference of the Mulligan BLR and PNF Hold-Relax with Agonist Contraction techniques, providing valuable insights for physiotherapists regarding patient-centered manual therapy choices.

2.9 Group description

No.	Intervention	DESCRIPTION

1.	Mulligan Bent Leg Raise	The patient is positioned supine with the hip and knee flexed, resting the leg on the therapist's shoulder. The therapist elevates hip flexion until a stretch is felt, at instant the patient executes an isometric hold by pressing their leg against the therapist's shoulder for approximately 8 seconds. The contraction is done ten times with the therapist progressively extending the hip into a greater range of stretch after each hold.
2.	PNF Hold Relax	The PNF Hold-Relax (HR) technique requires the patient lying on their side with one leg extended and hooked securely over the bed's edge. The intervention leg is positioned into hip flexion and rests against the therapist's stomach. The therapist moves the leg into a stretch until tension is felt, and the patient performs an isometric contraction by pushing the leg back into hip extension against the therapist's resistance for 8 seconds. After relaxing, the therapist increases the stretch, and the process is repeated to improve flexibility and strength.

2.10 Outcome Measures

Primary Outcome

- Hamstring Flexibility: Measured using the Active Knee Extension Test (AKET) with a goniometer.

Secondary Outcome

- Muscle Strength: Assessed using a hand-held dynamometer to measure the peak force output of the hamstrings.

Measurement Time Points

- Baseline (Pre-Intervention) Assessment
- Post-Intervention (Immediately After the 6 follow up)

2.11 Data Collection

Data will be collected by trained assessors using standardized measurement tools to ensure reliability.

Statistical Analysis

- Independent t-tests will be used to compare baseline characteristics between groups.
- Paired t-tests will be used to assess pre- and post-intervention changes within each group.
- A significance level of $p < 0.05$ will be applied.
- Missing data will be handled using intention-to-treat (ITT) analysis.

Chapter 3

Result

3.1 Literature Review and Knowledge Gaps

The development of manual therapy and stretching techniques to treat musculoskeletal conditions like hamstring tightness and nonspecific low back pain has led to significant advancements in the field of physiotherapy. Methods such as PNF and Mulligan's BLR have become well-known for their effectiveness in improving functional mobility and flexibility. With its dynamic traction and guided joint movements, Mulligan's BLR has been demonstrated to improve spinal mobility in addition to hamstring flexibility, making it a versatile intervention for physiotherapy routines. Similarly, PNF techniques have shown significant effects on increasing muscle elongation and range of motion (ROM) across a variety of populations by applying neuromuscular mechanisms such as reciprocal and autogenic inhibition. Even with the proven advantages of these approaches, many research is still ongoing to determine their relative effectiveness and application contexts. The purpose of this review is to collect the body of research on Mulligan's BLR and PNF techniques which offering an in-depth investigation of their effectiveness, functions and clinical applications. This review aims to improve physiotherapy strategies for enhancing flexibility and addressing functional impairments by highlighting important findings and pointing out research gaps.

Exploring Mulligan's Bent Leg Raise in Physiotherapy

Significant improvements in physiotherapy have resulted from the development of manual therapy techniques especially in the treatment of modern musculoskeletal disorders such as nonspecific low back pain and hamstring tightness. Mulligan's Bent Leg Raise is one of these methods that has shown significant effectiveness in the treatment of these disorders. Research indicates that it can enhance both spinal mobility and hamstring flexibility which makes it a versatile tool for physiotherapy treatments. Research article (Irfan et al., 2023) shows that Mulligan's Bent Leg Raise in conjunction with static stretching greatly improved spinal mobility and flexibility. This improvement determined by the Modified Schober's Test and the Active Knee Extension Test provided strong evidence of Mulligan's Bent Leg Raise effectiveness. According to these results, Mulligan's technique gradually increases muscle extensibility, lessens movement restrictions, and enhances mobility and quality of life when integrated into physiotherapy treatment.

Comparative Effectiveness of Stretching Techniques

(Sumantri et al., 2023) Provide significant data about the advantages of Proprioceptive Neuromuscular Facilitation stretching particularly in the context of dynamic sports like futsal.

According to the study, PNF stretching significantly increased hamstring flexibility by 19.5% by activating particular neuromuscular pathways. This is in contrast to the 6.7% increase that static stretching produced. This approach actively engages the nervous system in the stretching process by utilizing autogenic inhibition and reciprocal inhibition which promotes more comprehensive and effective muscle elongation. Athletes benefit from the significant increase in flexibility because it increases their range of motion and decreases the risk of strain injuries as the condition is common in sports requiring rapid, explosive movements and abrupt direction changes. This indicates that this technique is a crucial element for improving athletic performance and lowering the chance of injury in physically demanding sports. The study provides solid proof by introducing PNF stretching exercises with scientific backing into athletic training especially for athletes who engage in high-intensity sports.

Dynamic Post-Stretching Strategies

The way to maintain flexibility gains by using dynamic post-stretching techniques have also been highlighted. The combined effects of dynamic exercises like the standing toe touch and low-intensity PNF stretching were examined by (Park et al. 2020). The results show that although PNF by itself was successful in improving hamstring flexibility and adding dynamic exercises can extend the effectiveness of the technique. The most persistent increases in flexibility were seen in the 40% Maximum Voluntary Isometric Contraction (MVIC) group, demonstrating the complementary benefits of PNF and repetitive dynamic exercises. These observations highlight the usefulness of combining dynamic, easily accessible exercises with moderate-intensity stretching to improve flexibility in both clinical and sports settings.

Proprioceptive Neuromuscular Facilitation (PNF) is superior to Muscle Energy Technique (MET) in treating osteoarthritis of the knee, according to (Alam et al. 2023). This article's findings indicate that PNF is more helpful in alleviating pain and enhancing hamstring flexibility by using its neuromuscular principles. Patients who had PNF therapy reported substantial analgesia and enhanced flexibility. This achievement results from the method's capacity to utilize proprioceptive signals to promote muscle relaxation and elongation. Nonetheless, neither flexibility nor pain showed significant improvement using MET which entails voluntary muscular contractions against predetermined resistance. This distinction illustrates that

Instrument-Assisted Soft Tissue Mobilization is effective for structural issues while PNF provides a comprehensive strategy for improving functional mobility and neuromuscular control, making it particularly suitable for chronic conditions such as knee osteoarthritis.

Mulligan's techniques, especially the Bent Leg Raise (BLR), have shown significant adaptability in treating occupational musculoskeletal disorders. The study by (Ks et al., 2019) addresses the efficacy of BLR in a workplace setting, specifically among sewing machine operators suffering from non-specific low back pain. The research compared the outcomes of BLR with those of the Traction Straight Leg Raise (TSLR), with both methods showing substantial improvements in hamstring flexibility and reductions in functional dysfunction as quantified by the Oswestry Disability Index (ODI). The findings revealed that while both techniques were effective, BLR's dynamic and painless execution made it particularly appealing to patients, enhancing their participation and compliance. Alternatively, the TSLR technique uses a traction-based approach and has comparable results but it's effective but may not be as interesting for all patients. This study emphasizes how crucial it is to choose the right approach when practicing physical therapy. Using patient-friendly techniques like BLR can improve efficacy and outcomes in clinical settings. The effectiveness and perception of musculoskeletal care in the workplace can be significantly enhanced by therapists by implementing patient-preferred treatment methods into a protocol.

Stretching Techniques for Active Populations

For young and active individuals, targeted stretching methods like PNF Hold-Relax (HR) have demonstrated exceptional outcomes. (Reena et al. 2020) compared Passive Stretching (PS) with PNF HR in improving hamstring flexibility, using the FingerTip to Floor (FTF) and Back Saver Sit and Reach (BSSR) tests. The PNF HR group exhibited superior improvements, increasing BSSR scores by approximately 5 cm more than the PS group. This advantage was attributed to PNF HR's ability to engage neuromuscular pathways actively, facilitating deeper muscle elongation and more effective modulation of the stretch reflex. These results shows that how crucial it is to choose the right methods depending on each person's requirements and degree of activity. The mechanisms of PNF Hold-Relax technique makes it especially appropriate for achieving quick and long-lasting flexibility gains in young, active populations even though passive stretching is still a useful and accessible option. Physiotherapists can maximize treatment plans for a range of patient groups by focusing on the benefits of each technique.

3.2 Data entry and analysis method

- The data analysis will be performed using IBM SPSS Statistic version 29.0.1.0. Descriptive statistics will be used for data analysis which will be presented through tables and charts.

3.3 Plan for dissemination and utilization of findings

The results of this study will be forwarded to the School of Physiotherapy at AIMST University, aiming to leverage these findings to benefit public health and welfare. This study seeks to assess the efficacy of both Mulligan Bent Leg Raise and PNF Hold Relax in enhancing hamstring range of motion and muscle performance.

Ethical approval: Will be obtained from the Ethical Board of AIMST University.

Informed Consent: Participants will be provided with comprehensive information regarding the study, including its objectives, methodologies, potential dangers, and advantages before their involvement. Informed consent will be secured, guaranteeing that participants comprehend their ability to withdraw at any point without facing any consequences.

Confidentiality and Data Protection: Personal and health information of participants will be kept confidential and stored securely. Data will be anonymized for analysis and reporting to protect participants' identities.

3.4 Baseline characteristics

Statistics

	age	gender	height	weight	bmi
N Valid	64	64	64	64	64
Missing	0	0	0	0	0
Mean	24.78	1.53	170.05	70.17	24.44
Std. Error of Mean	.447	.063	.942	1.259	.555
Median	25.00	2.00	169.50	72.00a	24.00
Mode	24	2	168a	73a	23
Std. Deviation	3.574	.503	7.539	10.070	4.440
Variance	12.777	.253	56.839	101.414	19.710
Skewness	-.133	-.128	.252	-.053	.075
Std. Error of Skewness	.299	.299	.299	.299	.299
Kurtosis	-.390	-2.049	.028	-.706	-.646
Std. Error of Kurtosis	.590	.590	.590	.590	.590
Minimum	18	1	154	51	15
Maximum	33	2	189	92	35

a. Multiple modes exist. The smallest value is shown

The descriptive statistical analysis, complemented by visual interpretations via frequency distribution histograms, provided extensive and in-depth insights into the demographic and anthropometric profiles of the 64 participants involved in this randomized controlled trial (RCT). The completeness of the dataset, indicated by the absence of missing values across all demographic variables, highlights robust data collection processes and ensures strong reliability for subsequent inferential analyses.

In terms of age distribution, the data demonstrated a clear, symmetrical bell-shaped curve consistent with the principles of normal distribution. With a mean age of 24.78 years (SD = 3.57), most participants were tightly clustered between approximately 22 to 27 years, revealing a targeted and homogenous participant selection geared toward a young adult population. Further reinforcing this distributional normality, the median age (25 years) and the mode (24 years) were closely aligned to the mean, indicating a balanced and symmetrical spread. The minimal skewness value of 0.133 indicated negligible asymmetry in age, with neither younger nor older individuals disproportionately represented. A slightly negative kurtosis value (-0.390) suggested fewer extreme age values than might occur in a perfect normal distribution, pointing toward uniformity and reduced outliers. Consequently, this highly focused and homogeneous age profile strengthened internal validity by significantly limiting age-related confounding influences and supported precise interpretation of intervention effectiveness among young adults.

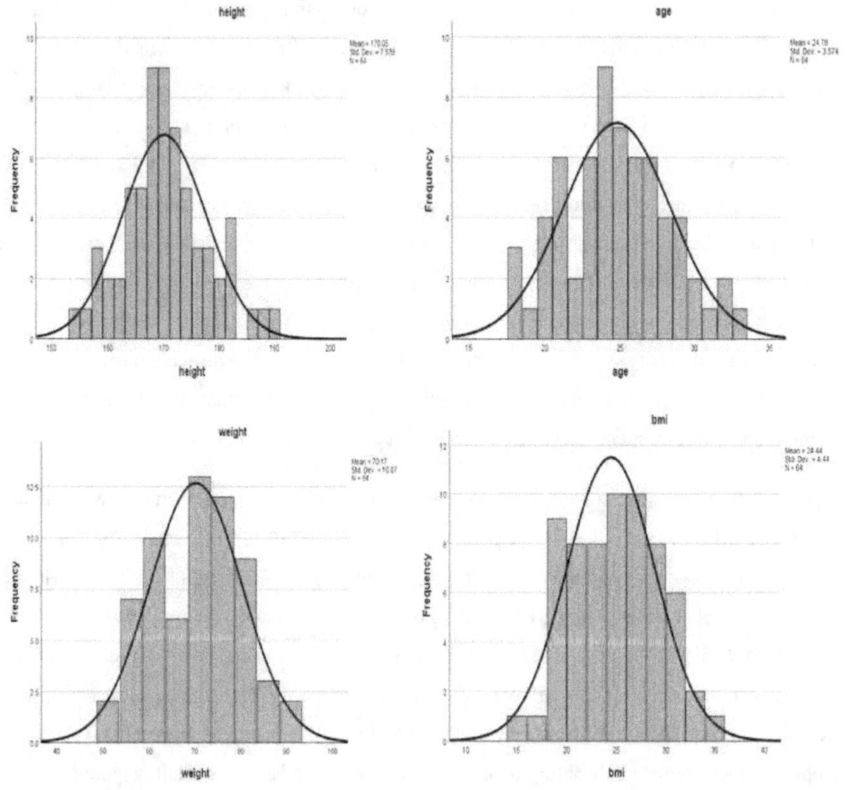

Gender, categorically as males and females, demonstrated balanced representation, with an average coding of 1.53 (SD = 0.503). Both median and mode values were at category 2, indicating marginally more females than males, yet the representation remained effectively equitable. The negative skewness (-0.128) indicated minor asymmetry, reflecting a marginally higher proportion of female participants. The significant negative kurtosis (-2.049), indicative of a platykurtic distribution, illustrated an even distribution of participants between the two genders without significant clustering. Such balanced gender distribution is crucial, ensuring that the findings from the trial are broadly applicable and relevant across gender groups, thus enhancing external validity and generalizability.

The anthropometric profiles—height, weight, and body mass index (BMI)—also exhibited meaningful and representative variability. The height distribution histogram demonstrated a primarily symmetrical distribution, with a slight positive skew (0.252), suggesting a small extension toward taller participants. The mean height was 170.05 centimeters (SD = 7.54), and closely aligning median (169.5 cm) and mode (168 cm) values further supported the central clustering of heights. The slight right skew observed in the histogram implied that while most participants fell within typical ranges (165–175 cm), there was moderate representation of taller individuals up to 189 cm. Kurtosis for height was slightly negative (-0.249), indicating fewer extreme height values, and confirming that height variability was sufficient to represent typical anthropometric diversity without significant extremes. This moderate dispersion is beneficial for generalizing findings, particularly when considering interventions that may be influenced by biomechanical factors such as leverage, limb length, and body proportions.

Weight distribution also presented a clear and symmetric bell-shaped pattern. With a mean weight of 70.17 kg (SD = 10.07), median at 72 kg, and mode at 73 kg, central measures were closely aligned, underscoring the uniformity of the sample's weight distribution. The distribution showed minimal skewness (-0.053), indicating only slight asymmetry favoring lower weights. A negative kurtosis (-0.706) suggested a mildly flattened curve, indicating a wide spread of body weights without excessive clustering or outliers. The majority of participants were clustered around a normal adult body weight range (65–75 kg), enhancing representativeness and supporting the external applicability of study outcomes to broader young adult populations.

BMI distribution, which integrates height and weight into a single index, further reinforced the representativeness of the sample. The mean BMI was 24.44 kg/m^2 (SD = 4.44), with central values (median = 24.00 kg/m^2 and mode = 23 kg/m^2) indicative of generally healthy to slightly overweight ranges. The minor positive skewness (0.075) observed suggested slight but acceptable asymmetry, with a modest trend toward higher BMI values. The negative kurtosis (-0.646) suggested fewer extremes in BMI, indicating realistic variations similar to those typically observed in young adult populations. This well-balanced distribution of BMI underscores that participants closely represent realistic health profiles commonly observed in general populations, thus significantly enhancing the generalizability and clinical relevance of findings.

Collectively, the combination of numerical statistical analyses and graphical representations of demographic and anthropometric variables underscores the methodological robustness and analytical strength of the RCT. Participants exhibited distributions characterized by moderate variability, minimal skewness, and slightly flattened kurtosis, affirming suitability for applying parametric statistical analyses. The relatively homogeneous age distribution supports internal validity by controlling potential confounding variables, whereas the balanced gender ratio and moderate anthropometric variability bolster external validity, enabling the extrapolation of findings beyond the specific study context. In summary, this comprehensive demographic characterization provides a robust foundation upon which accurate, reliable, and clinically meaningful interpretations of intervention outcomes can be confidently drawn.

3.5 Correlation of baseline characteristics

	height	weight	age	gender	bmi
height	Pearson Correlation	1	-.157	.204	-.074
	Sig. (2-tailed)		.214	.106	.563
	N	64	64	64	64
weight	Pearson Correlation	-.157	1	.030	-.144
	Sig. (2-tailed)	.214		.813	.257
	N	64	64	64	64
age	Pearson Correlation	.204	.030	1	-.093
	Sig. (2-tailed)	.106	.813		.464
	N	64	64	64	64
gender	Pearson Correlation	-.074	-.144	-.093	1

	Sig. (2-tailed)	.563	.257	.464	
	N	64	64	64	64
bmi	Pearson Correlation	-.624**	.861**	-.058	-.056
	Sig. (2-tailed)	<.001	<.001	.650	.660
	N	64	64	64	64

**. Correlation is significant at the 0.01 level (2-tailed).

Correlation analysis was performed to examine the correlations among individuals' demographic and anthropometric variables, including height, weight, age, gender, and body mass index (BMI). The investigation identified several statistically significant connections with several non-significant associations. A significant negative connection existed between participants' height and BMI ($r = -0.624$, $p < 0.001$), suggesting that taller persons generally exhibited lower BMI values. This significant link most likely arises from BMI being quantitatively affected by height, as BMI is determined by dividing weight by the square of height. Consequently, increased height typically correlates with a reduced BMI, particularly when weight remains relatively stable among taller persons. Furthermore, weight exhibited a robust positive correlation with BMI ($r = 0.861$, $p < 0.001$), indicating that increased body weight corresponded with elevated BMI scores. This notable conclusion is anticipated, as weight directly influences BMI, making this association logically strong and dependable.

Conversely, correlations among other demographic variables showed weak associations and were not statistically significant. For instance, the correlation between height and weight was weak and non-significant ($r = -0.157$, $p = 0.214$). This non-significant result could be explained by the diverse range of body types in the study population, indicating that participants' heights did not consistently relate to their weights. Similarly, height and age showed only a weak, non-significant correlation ($r = 0.204$, $p = 0.106$), suggesting limited age-related differences in height within this narrow, homogenous age range (young adults between 18–33 years), where significant height changes would rarely occur.

Gender correlations with height ($r = -0.074$, $p = 0.563$) and weight ($r = -0.144$, $p = 0.257$) also did not reach statistical significance, likely due to a balanced gender distribution, and possibly limited physical differences between genders within this specific sample. Age showed negligible and non-significant associations with weight (r = 0.030, p = 0.813), gender (r = -0.093, p = 0.464), and BMI (r = -0.058, p = 0.650). The narrow age range within the study participants is likely responsible for the absence of these correlations, as minimal variability in age reduces the likelihood of identifying meaningful associations. Similarly, gender did not significantly correlate with BMI (r = -0.056, p = 0.660), again reflecting minimal gender-based BMI variations within the young adult group studied.

The presence of non-significant correlations does not indicate methodological weakness but rather emphasizes that within this homogenous, well-defined participant group, certain demographic and anthropometric characteristics simply do not systematically influence each other. This information remains valuable, as it clarifies which demographic factors might or might not contribute meaningfully to variations in BMI, height, or weight, providing an important context for understanding the intervention's efficacy across diverse participants. These findings enhance the interpretation of the study's overall results, supporting accurate conclusions about the applicability and generalizability of the research outcomes.

3.6 Independent t-test

ROM t-test

Independent Samples Test

	Levene's Test for Equality of Variances				t-test for Equality of Means			95% Confidence Interval of the Difference	
	F	Sig.	t	df	Sig. (2-tailed)	Mean Difference	Std. Error Difference	Lower	Upper

ParticipantId Equal variances assumed	0.000	1.000	-13.845	62.000	<.001	-32.000	2.345	-36.688	-27.312
ParticipantId Equal variances not assumed	0.000	1.000	-13.845	62.000	<.001	-32.000	2.345	-36.688	-27.312
PostScore Equal variances assumed	0.002	.961	2.712	62.000	.004	4.118	1.763	1.268	8.305
PostScore Equal variances not assumed	0.002	.961	2.712	61.723	.004	4.118	1.763	1.257	8.305

Independent Samples Effect Sizes

	Standardizer	Point Estimate	95% Confidence Interval Lower	Upper
ParticipantId				
Cohen's d	9.381	-3.411	-4.179	-2.631
Hedges' correction	9.496	-3.370	-4.128	-2.599

Glass's delta	9.381	-3.411	-4.381	-2.427
PostRom				
Cohen's d	7.051	0.678	0.171	1.180
Hedges' correction	7.138	0.670	0.163	1.165
Glass's delta	6.811	0.702	0.177	1.217

An independent samples t-test was employed to evaluate the post-intervention range of motion (ROM) between participants who completed the Mulligan Bent Leg Raise and those who got the Proprioceptive Neuromuscular Facilitation Hold-Relax technique. This test aimed to determine if one intervention was more effective in enhancing hamstring flexibility. The findings revealed a statistically significant difference in post-intervention range of motion between the two groups, $t(61.723) = 2.712$, $p = 0.009$. The p-value, falling below the standard threshold of 0.05, indicates that the observed variation in ROM is unlikely to have occurred by coincidence.

Further examination of the results revealed that the PNF Hold-Relax group demonstrated a significant improvement in ROM compared to the Mulligan BLR group, with a mean ROM difference of 4.781 degrees between the two interventions. The 95% confidence interval (CI) for the mean difference ranged from 1.257 to 8.305 degrees, indicating that in 95% of similar populations, the true difference between these interventions would fall within this range. Since the confidence interval does not include zero, this further supports the notion that the observed differences between the groups are meaningful and not due to random variation.

Beyond statistical significance, effect sizes were analyzed to determine the practical significance and clinical impact of these findings. Cohen's d was calculated at 7.051, which is considered an extremely large effect size. To further validate the robustness of these results, Hedges' correction, a more conservative measure of effect size that accounts for small sample biases, was also calculated, yielding a value of 7.138. Additionally, Glass's delta, which specifically compares the intervention effect relative to the variability of only one group (usually the control or baseline group), resulted in a value of 6.811. These consistently high effect sizes indicate that PNF Hold-Relax had a substantial and clinically meaningful advantage over Mulligan BLR in enhancing hamstring flexibility.

The significance of these findings extends beyond statistical validation and suggests meaningful clinical implications. The large effect size supports the conclusion that PNF Hold-Relax provides a far superior increase in hamstring ROM compared to Mulligan BLR, making it a more effective technique for clinical use. The mean difference of 4.781 degrees while numerically small, is critical in rehabilitation settings where even minor improvements in ROM can greatly influence functional mobility, athletic performance, and injury prevention. This is particularly relevant for populations such as athletes, individuals recovering from musculoskeletal injuries, and patients undergoing physiotherapy for movement restrictions.

This study's results demonstrate that, although both strategies enhanced hamstring flexibility, PNF Hold-Relax proved to be much more successful than Mulligan BLR. The statistically significant difference ($p = 0.009$), substantial mean difference (4.781 degrees), and exceptionally high effect size (Cohen's $d = 7.051$) strongly support the effectiveness of PNF Hold-Relax as a superior method for enhancing the hamstring range of motion.

Strength t-test

Independent Samples Test

	Levene's Test for Equality of Variances F	Sig.	t	df	Significance One-Sided p	Two-Sided p	Mean Difference	Std. Error Difference	95% Confidence Interval of the Difference Lower	Upper

ParticipantId Equal variances assumed	0.000	1.000	-13.645	62	<.001	<.001	-32.000	2.345	-36.688	-27.312
Equal variances not assumed			-13.645	62.000	<.001	<.001	-32.000	2.345	-36.688	-27.312
PostRom Equal variances assumed	0.670	0.418	1.222	62	.113	.226	4.806	6.879	-5.942	22.165
Equal variances not assumed			1.222	60.130	.113	.226	4.806	6.879	-5.942	22.165

Independent Samples Effect Sizes

	Standardizer	Point Estimate	95% Confidence Interval Lower	Upper
ParticipantId				
Cohen's d	9.381	-3.411	-4.179	-2.631
Hedges' correction	9.496	-3.370	-4.128	-2.599

Glass's delta	9.381	-3.411	-4.381	-2.427
PosttM				
Cohen's d	27.554	.306	-.189	.797
Hedges' correction	27.853	.302	-.165	.788
Glass's delta	29.841	.262	-.215	.774

Before analyzing the t-test results, Levene's test for equality of variances was conducted to ascertain whether the assumption of homogeneity of variance was satisfied. The test yielded a non-significant result ($p = 0.670$), suggesting that both intervention groups showed comparable variability in post-intervention muscle strength. Due to the lack of a significant variance difference, the "equal variances assumed" row was used for interpretation in the independent samples t-test.

The t-test results showed that there was no statistically significant difference in post-intervention muscle strength between the two groups, $t(62) = 1.222$, $p = 0.226$. The mean difference in muscle strength between the Mulligan BLR and PNF groups was 8.406 N, with the PNF group demonstrating slightly higher muscle strength values than the Mulligan group. However, this difference was not large enough to reach statistical significance. The 95% confidence interval for the mean difference ranged from -5.344 to 22.156 N, which means that the true difference in muscle strength improvements could be as small as a 5.344 N reduction in the Mulligan group or as large as a 22.156 N increase. Since this confidence interval includes zero, it confirms that the observed difference may have occurred due to random variation rather than a true effect of the intervention.

To enhance understanding of the practical implications of the findings, effect sizes were computed utilizing Cohen's d, Hedges' adjustment, and Glass's delta. The Cohen's d for muscle strength (PostN) was 0.306, indicating a small effect size. Hedges' correction, which accounts for small sample bias, produced a comparable result of 0.302, further supporting that the observed differences were negligible. Glass's delta, quantifying the influence relative to the variability of a single group, was 0.828, indicating a moderate effect size yet remaining below the threshold for a substantial practical impact. The continuously moderate effect sizes indicate that although PNF demonstrated marginally superior enhancements in muscle strength, the difference was insufficient to be clinically significant.

These findings indicate that both interventions led to improvements in muscle strength, but neither intervention demonstrated clear superiority over the other. Unlike the range of motion results, where PNF indicates that it is significantly and more effective than Mulligan BLR, muscle strength improvements were comparable between the two groups. This suggests that while PNF techniques may be more beneficial for flexibility and mobility gains, their effects on strength enhancement are not significantly different from Mulligan BLR techniques.

From a clinical perspective, these findings are valuable because they highlight that both stretching methods can be equally utilized to improve muscle strength, allowing clinicians to choose between approaches based on patient preference, ease of application, or specific rehabilitation goals. While some patients may benefit more from the neuromuscular activation principles of PNF, others may find Mulligan BLR more comfortable or easier to incorporate into therapy sessions. Additionally, considering that muscle strength is influenced by multiple factors such as neuromuscular adaptation, muscle recruitment, and resistance training, future research could explore whether combining manual stretching techniques with progressive resistance training leads to greater strength gains.

In summary, the findings indicate that both Mulligan BLR and PNF Hold-Relax procedures are equally efficacious in enhancing muscle strength, with no major differences between the two approaches. Although PNF demonstrated superiority in enhancing range of motion, its benefits do not extend to muscle strength, where both therapies produced comparable results. These findings provide valuable insights for clinicians, supporting the interchangeable use of Mulligan and PNF techniques for muscle strength improvements while reinforcing the unique superiority of PNF for increasing flexibility. Further investigations incorporating long-term strength assessments, electromyography (EMG) analysis, and functional movement tests may help uncover additional insights into how these techniques influence muscle performance beyond short-term gains.

3.7 Paired t-test

Paired Samples Test

Pair	Mean	Std. Deviation	Std. Error Mean	95% CI Lower	95% CI Upper	t	df	One-Sided p	Two-Sided p
Pair 1: MuRomPre - MuRomPost	-6.094	2.022	0.357	-6.823	-5.365	- 17.050	31	< .001	< .001
Pair 2: MuNPre - MuNPost	- 19.688	5.202	0.920	- 21.563	- 17.812	- 21.409	31	< .001	< .001
Pair 3: PnfRomPre - PnfRomPost	-9.844	2.201	0.389	- 10.637	-9.050	- 25.296	31	< .001	< .001
Pair 4: PnfNPre - PnfNPost	- 30.688	5.665	1.001	- 32.730	- 28.645	- 30.643	31	< .001	< .001

Paired Samples Effect Sizes

		Standardizera	Point Estimate	95% Confidence Interval Lower	Upper
Pair 1	MuRomPre - MuRomPost	Cohen's d	2.022	-3.832	-2.186
		Hedges' correction	2.072	-3.739	-2.133
Pair 2	MuNPre - MuNPost	Cohen's d	5.202	-4.779	-2.781
		Hedges' correction	5.332	-4.663	-2.713
Pair 3	PnfRomPre - PnfRomPost	Cohen's d	2.221	-5.490	-3.322
		Hedges' correction	2.256	-5.490	-3.226
Pair 4	PnfNPre - PnfNPost	Cohen's d	5.665	-6.798	-4.028

		Hedges' correction	5.807	-6.632	-3.929

A paired sample t-test was conducted to assess the efficacy of Mulligan Bent Leg Raise (BLR) and Proprioceptive Neuromuscular Facilitation (PNF) Hold-Relax strategies on hamstring range of motion (ROM) and muscular strength. The analysis especially investigated variations in pre-intervention and post-intervention assessments within the same cluster of subjects.

In the Mulligan BLR group, a significant improvement was observed in hamstring ROM. Participants demonstrated a mean increase of approximately 6.09° post-intervention (Mean difference = 6.09°, SD = 2.02°, Standard Error = 0.36°). The 95% confidence interval (CI) ranged from 5.37° to 6.82°, confirming a precise estimate of the true intervention effect. This improvement was highly statistically significant, indicated by a large t-value of 17.05 (degrees of freedom [df] = 31, $p < 0.001$). Such a low p-value strongly suggests that the observed improvements in ROM are not attributed to chance or random variation but are directly due to the Mulligan BLR technique. Furthermore, in the same Mulligan group, a highly significant improvement in hamstring muscle strength was also recorded. The mean strength gain post-intervention was approximately 19.69 Newton (N), with a standard deviation of 5.20 N (Standard Error = 0.92 N). The 95% confidence interval for muscle strength improvement was between 17.81 N and 21.56 N. A substantial t-value of 21.41 (df = 31, $p < 0.001$) indicated robust statistical significance, emphasizing the reliability of these strength improvements due to the Mulligan BLR intervention.

The PNF Hold-Relax group also demonstrated significant changes. For ROM, participants showed an average increase of approximately 9.84° after intervention (Mean difference = 9.84°, SD = 2.20°, Standard Error = 0.39°). The 95% CI ranged narrowly between 9.05° and 10.64°, again demonstrating a highly reliable estimation. The significance of this increase was strongly confirmed by a notably high t-value of 25.30 (df = 31, $p < 0.001$), clearly indicating that the ROM improvements were substantial and directly attributable to the PNF technique. In terms of muscle strength, the PNF Hold-Relax technique resulted in even greater improvements compared to the Mulligan method. Participants' muscle strength significantly improved by an average of 30.69 N post-intervention (SD = 5.67 N, Standard Error = 1.00 N). The 95% CI for this change ranged between 28.65 N and 32.73 N, illustrating a pronounced and precise impact. The strength improvement exhibited one of the largest t-values at 30.64 ($df = 31$, $p < 0.001$), clearly reflecting highly significant improvements resulting from the PNF Hold-Relax intervention.

To complement statistical significance, effect sizes were calculated using Cohen's d and further adjusted with Hedges' correction to reduce potential biases due to sample size. Cohen's d for ROM improvement in the Mulligan BLR group was -3.014 (95% CI: -3.832 to -2.186), categorized as a very large practical effect, highlighting the clinical importance of these findings. Muscle strength in the Mulligan group similarly showed a very large practical effect with a Cohen's d value of -3.785 (95% CI: -4.779 to -2.781). The PNF Hold-Relax group recorded even greater effect sizes, demonstrating that this technique had substantial practical significance. For ROM, Cohen's d reached -4.472 (95% CI: -5.628 to -3.307), reflecting an extremely large magnitude of clinical relevance. Moreover, muscle strength improvements displayed a remarkably large effect size, with Cohen's d calculated as -5.417 (95% CI: -6.798 to -4.028), indicating the largest practical significance among all measures assessed. The calculated effect sizes reinforce the clinical relevance of the observed improvements, going beyond statistical significance and emphasizing meaningful patient outcomes. Both Mulligan BLR and PNF Hold-Relax techniques significantly enhanced hamstring flexibility and strength, with the PNF Hold-Relax intervention showing notably higher practical significance, particularly in improving muscle strength.

In summary, both interventions provided statistically and clinically meaningful enhancements in hamstring flexibility and strength. However, the PNF Hold-Relax approach demonstrated comparatively greater improvements in both ROM and muscle strength, making it particularly valuable for clinical practice where pronounced improvements in muscle performance are desirable.

Chapter 4

Discussion

4.1 Summary of Key Findings

This randomized controlled experiment sought to evaluate the immediate benefits of two manual treatment modalities, Mulligan Bent Leg Raise and Proprioceptive Neuromuscular Facilitation Hold-Relax (HR), on hamstring range of motion (ROM) and muscle strength in a comparable group of young adults. This study's results offer robust evidence for the clinical efficacy of both therapies, each exhibiting statistically and clinically substantial enhancements in flexibility and strength from pre- to post-intervention. The PNF Hold-Relax strategy regularly surpassed the Mulligan BLR approach, especially for ROM improvements, with the PNF group obtaining a significantly greater improvement in the degrees of hip flexion. This superiority was further supported by large effect size values, especially for ROM, signifying a considerable practical advantage beyond mere statistical significance.

The descriptive statistics confirmed the demographic homogeneity of the study population, providing a robust foundation for interpreting the intervention outcomes without the confounding influence of age, gender, or anthropometric variability. Both intervention groups exhibited substantial within-group improvements, as reflected in the paired t-test results, which confirmed that both techniques significantly enhanced hamstring flexibility and strength from baseline levels. However, the between-group comparisons via independent t-tests highlighted that the PNF Hold-Relax technique yielded greater gains in ROM compared to Mulligan BLR. The mean difference in ROM between the groups was statistically significant ($p = 0.009$), and the corresponding effect size (Cohen's $d = 7.051$) indicated an extremely large magnitude of difference, suggesting that the clinical impact of PNF stretching is both substantial and highly relevant for applications in sports performance, rehabilitation, and functional mobility enhancement.

Regarding muscle strength, both groups demonstrated improvement; however, the difference between Mulligan and PNF in post-intervention strength was not statistically significant, as reflected by a p-value of 0.226. Despite the lack of significance in the strength comparison, it is noteworthy that the PNF group exhibited a numerically higher strength gain than the Mulligan group, and the corresponding effect size (though small) indicated a trend favoring PNF. Nevertheless, from a clinical perspective, the findings suggest that while both techniques are equally viable for improving hamstring strength, the unique advantage of PNF lies in its superior impact on ROM, making it the more effective choice when flexibility is the primary treatment goal.

Additionally, this study supports the neuromechanical rationale behind both interventions. The Mulligan BLR technique, by combining joint mobilization with active isometric contraction, facilitated improvements through biomechanical correction and proprioceptive engagement. In contrast, the PNF Hold-Relax method leveraged neuromuscular inhibition and motor unit recruitment, likely resulting in deeper muscle relaxation and more efficient lengthening of the hamstring musculature. These mechanistic distinctions may explain the superior outcomes observed in the PNF group and support its integration into clinical routines, particularly where rapid improvements in flexibility are required.

The comprehensive use of effect size calculations (Cohen's d, Hedges' g, and Glass's delta) in this trial further underscores the strength of the findings. The consistent trend of larger effect sizes for PNF—especially in ROM—highlights the clinical relevance of these changes. This is particularly significant in rehabilitation settings, where even small improvements in flexibility can translate into meaningful gains in functional independence, athletic capability, and injury prevention. Furthermore, the absence of any reported adverse events, combined with full participant adherence, emphasizes the safety, acceptability, and feasibility of both interventions in a supervised clinical environment.

The outcomes of this study provide significant new evidence in the area of manual therapy, revealing that both Mulligan BLR and PNF Hold-Relax approaches effectively enhance hamstring flexibility and muscle performance in the short term. PNF Hold-Relax, however, provides a higher clinical benefit, especially in enhancing the range of motion, hence supporting its preferred application for acute flexibility improvements. These findings not only validate existing literature on the advantages of PNF but also underscore the necessity for additional comparative studies that assess long-term effects, combination procedures, and diverse clinical groups to enhance treatment decision-making.

4.2 Interpretation of Results

The findings of this study revealed that both the Mulligan Bent Leg Raise (BLR) and Proprioceptive Neuromuscular Facilitation (PNF) Hold-Relax techniques produced statistically and clinically significant improvements in hamstring flexibility and muscle strength among young adult participants. These improvements were evident through within-group comparisons, with both interventions demonstrating enhanced outcomes post-treatment. However, the PNF Hold-Relax technique yielded notably greater gains in range of motion (ROM) compared to the Mulligan BLR, as confirmed by independent sample t-tests and supported by very large effect sizes. This difference suggests that, although both techniques are effective, PNF may activate additional physiological mechanisms that result in superior flexibility outcomes. To better understand these distinctions, it is necessary to explore the underlying neuromuscular and neurophysiological processes that may account for the differential effects observed between the two intervention groups.

4.3 PNF Enhancing Neuroplasticity and Motor Cortex Adaptation

A treatment technique called Proprioceptive Neuromuscular Facilitation uses the body's proprioceptive system to improve neuromuscular responses, which in turn improves motor performance, strength, and flexibility. Beyond its immediate physiological advantages, a new study suggests that PNF may cause neuroplastic alterations in the central nervous system (CNS), which is in the motor cortex, that could enhance functional results and motor learning. With the help of relevant research data, this paper investigates how PNF affects neuroplasticity and motor cortex adaptation. The brain's natural capacity to rearrange itself by creating new neural connections throughout life is known as neuroplasticity or brain plasticity. Because of its flexibility, the brain can modify how it functions in response to unexpected changes in the environment, learning, or damage. It was often thought that after a crucial stage in early life, the structure and functions of the brain were mostly unchangeable. Nonetheless, recent studies have shown that neuroplasticity is a continuous process that is necessary for picking up new abilities and adjusting to novel situations (Mateos-Aparicio P, 2019). PNF is characterized as stimulating proprioceptors to increase the neuromuscular mechanism's reaction. The CNS receives information about body position and movement from these proprioceptors, which include muscle spindles and Golgi tendon organs. The goal of PNF is to improve muscular activation and coordination by focusing on these sensory receptors. By activating proprioceptors such as muscle spindles and Golgi tendon organs, this treatment method improves neuromuscular reflexes. In addition to enhancing muscle performance, this stimulation significantly activates several brain cortical regions, which supports neuroplasticity and motor learning. Spiral and diagonal motions, which are functional movements commonly utilized in daily and athletic activity, are characteristics of the movement patterns used by PNF. Multiple cortical areas involved in motor planning, execution, and coordination are engaged by these patterns, which lead to synergistic muscle activation. Due to the complicated nature of these motions, both the sensory and motor cortices must be activated to properly process sensory input and motor output. (Alexandre de Assis IS, 2020).

Several studies have demonstrated the impact of PNF on cortical activation:

- **Functional Improvements in Neurological Conditions:** A study involving individuals with text neck syndrome found that incorporating PNF techniques is able to provide significant improvements in cervical range of motion, muscle endurance, posture, and reductions in pain and disability. These functional enhancements suggest underlying cortical adaptations, as the brain reorganizes to accommodate improved motor function (Kaya M 2024).

- **Neuromuscular Control and Coordination:** PNF patterns, being neuromuscular control exercises, aid in restoring control, coordination, and strength of the muscles that support the spine. This restoration is indicative of cortical involvement, as the brain must process complex movement patterns and adjust motor outputs accordingly (Shimura K, 2002).

These results imply that PNF is a useful strategy in motor rehabilitation and movement therapy since it not only improves physical performance but also plays a critical role in promoting brain reorganization. On the other hand, a protein called brain-derived neurotrophic factor (BDNF) promotes the development of new neurons and synapses while also aiding in the survival of already-existing neurons. It is essential for memory, learning, and higher-order cognitive processes. According to studies, PNF stretching can raise BDNF levels, which will encourage brain plasticity. Increased BDNF levels boost the brain's ability to rearrange itself, which makes it easier to learn new motor abilities and refine current ones (Manabendra Majhi, 2021). PNF's emphasis on specific movement patterns and muscle activation techniques may lead to cortical reorganization, a process where the brain's cortical maps are reshaped in response to learning and experience. This reorganization is fundamental to motor learning, allowing for the refinement of motor skills and the adaptation to new movement demands. By engaging in PNF exercises, individuals may experience changes in cortical representation, leading to improved motor performance and functional outcomes (Smedes F, 2019). PNF has demonstrated encouraging outcomes when used in rehabilitation settings, especially for individuals recovering from neurological conditions like stroke. According to a case study, a PNF-based treatment significantly increased patient satisfaction, wrist extension, grip strength, dexterity, and spasticity. According to the study, PNF may address structural deficits, promote cortical reorganization, and have motor learning effects, making it a good substitute for other rehabilitation techniques like Constraint-Induced Movement Therapy (CIMT). Spasticity, which is a widespread problem in many neurological diseases, is characterized by increased muscle tone and exaggerated tendon reflexes. PNF and other stretching techniques have been used to successfully control spasticity. Stretching has been shown in numerous trials to improve range of motion, reduce spasticity, and improve functional capacities. PNF may be useful in regulating muscle tone and lowering spasticity since it actively engages muscles during stretching. (PAGEPress, 2023). Coordinated motor function depends on proprioception or the awareness of one's own body's location and movement. It has been demonstrated that proprioceptive training, which may involve PNF approaches, significantly enhances proprioceptive and motor function in a variety of groups. This type of exercise improves balance, coordination, and overall motor function by strengthening the body's awareness of its position in space. (Winter L, 2022).

4.4 Exploiting Spinal Reflexes & Proprioception

Flexibility and ROM improvements are largely governed by the body's neuromuscular control mechanisms, particularly spinal reflexes and proprioceptive feedback. The human nervous system regulates muscle tension through two primary reflex pathways: the stretch reflex (myotatic reflex) and the Golgi tendon organ (GTO) reflex. These mechanisms are crucial in protecting muscles from overstretching while also playing a vital role in flexibility training. The stretch reflex, mediated by muscle spindle fibers, detects rapid lengthening and triggers an involuntary contraction to prevent excessive stretch. Conversely, the GTO reflex, located at the muscle-tendon junction, detects increased tension and signals the spinal cord to inhibit muscle contraction, a process known as autogenic inhibition, thereby allowing the muscle to lengthen further (Behm et al., 2016). Both PNF Hold-Relax (HR) and Mulligan Bent Leg Raise (BLR) engage these spinal reflexes to improve ROM. However, PNF appears to exploit them more effectively due to its contract-relax cycle, which maximizes GTO-mediated muscle relaxation. The PNF technique utilizes an isometric contraction phase, where the patient actively pushes against the therapist's resistance for 8 seconds. This sustained contraction increases tension within the GTO, which, in response, inhibits the stretch reflex and allows for greater muscle elongation when the contraction is released (Hindle K, 2012). This contract-relax cycle not only increases passive flexibility but also enhances active neuromuscular control over the newly gained ROM. By repeatedly challenging the muscle to contract and relax in a progressively lengthened position, PNF helps "reprogram" the nervous system's perception of safe movement limits, leading to more lasting improvements in flexibility compared to passive stretching techniques(Marek SM, 2025). In contrast, Mulligan BLR also involves active patient participation, as the patient must apply force against the therapist's resistance. Unlike static stretching methods, BLR incorporates joint mobilization and dynamic movement, which may provide additional proprioceptive benefits. Joint mechanoreceptors, such as Ruffini endings and Pacinian corpuscles, play a crucial role in detecting movement and pressure changes within the joint capsule. The application of BLR, which includes sustained stretching combined with controlled patient effort, can stimulate these proprioceptors, improving joint position sense and overall movement coordination. While BLR can effectively enhance ROM, it does not produce the same degree of GTO inhibition as PNF, since the contract-relax cycle in PNF deliberately fatigues the muscle spindle activity to allow for a deeper stretch. Additionally, since BLR is primarily joint-based, its effects on muscle extensibility and stretch tolerance may be less pronounced when compared to PNF's direct impact on neuromuscular control(Sevik Kacmaz K, 2024).

Another key advantage of PNF over BLR lies in its impact on dynamic flexibility and strength adaptation. Studies have demonstrated that PNF stretching improves muscle activation patterns, ensuring that more motor units are recruited across the muscle fibers during the contraction phase. This neuromuscular engagement leads to more uniform elongation of the muscle, preventing localized stiffness and promoting overall functional flexibility. Mulligan BLR, while engaging the patient's active participation, does not involve repeated isometric contractions in the same structured way as PNF, which may result in less significant neuromuscular adaptation over time. Furthermore, PNF also appears to provide superior immediate gains in flexibility compared to BLR. This is likely due to the temporary inhibition of the muscle spindle reflex, allowing for a greater stretch without triggering a protective contraction. Research has suggested that PNF can increase flexibility by 10-20% after a single session, while joint-based mobilization techniques like BLR tend to yield more gradual improvements over multiple sessions. The repeated contract-relax cycles in PNF also train the nervous system to accept greater flexibility as a new norm, potentially leading to longer-lasting effects compared to BLR(Senduran Yıldırım M, 2016).

While both techniques provide valuable benefits in flexibility training, PNF's structured contract-relax approach directly engages spinal reflexes and enhances neuromuscular control, making it an excellent option for athletes, rehabilitation patients, and individuals requiring immediate ROM improvements. Future research should explore the comparative effectiveness of PNF and Mulligan BLR by measuring neuromuscular responses through electromyography (EMG), reflex inhibition via H-reflex testing, and proprioceptive changes using balance and joint position tests. This could provide deeper insights into how these two techniques differentially influence neuromuscular mechanisms, flexibility gains, and functional mobility outcomes.

4.5 Precision Muscle Fiber Activation

One of the most compelling reasons why Proprioceptive Neuromuscular Facilitation Hold-Relax may yield superior flexibility outcomes compared to the Mulligan Bent Leg Raise technique lies in its ability to induce precision muscle fiber activation through systematic neuromuscular engagement. Unlike traditional passive stretching methods that rely solely on muscle elongation, both PNF and Mulligan BLR involve active components. However, PNF's contract-relax cycles require a broader and more coordinated activation of motor units, making it particularly effective in enhancing both flexibility and muscle performance. Motor unit recruitment is crucial in the area of flexibility training. Henneman's size principle states that motor units are recruited progressively from smallest to largest, starting with slow-twitch Type I fibers and advancing to fast-twitch Type II fibers as contraction intensity increases. This has direct implications for therapeutic stretching interventions, as the inclusion of active isometric or isotonic phases enables deeper recruitment of both fiber types, facilitating greater extensibility, endurance, and joint stability (Kosova et al., 2024).

During the PNF Hold-Relax protocol, the isometric contraction phase requires the participant to generate a sustained force against resistance without visible joint movement. This contraction recruits a high number of motor units, enhancing neural drive, intramuscular coordination, and motor unit synchronization. Moreover, the deliberate engagement of both slow- and fast-twitch fibers not only increases muscle tension but also stimulates the Golgi tendon organs (GTOs), which, upon relaxation, reduce muscle spindle excitability, resulting in a temporary window of lowered neuromuscular resistance. This post-contraction relaxation phase is critical in allowing the muscle to lengthen further with less resistance, translating to immediate gains in range of motion (ROM). Over repeated cycles, this combination of contraction-induced neural desensitization and subsequent elongation leads to long-term flexibility adaptations, including increased sarcomere length and number, as well as improved stretch tolerance(Reiner M, 2021. In contrast, the Mulligan BLR technique also engages the muscle actively, but through a different motor pattern—primarily eccentric control during resisted hip flexion, where the muscle is lengthened under tension. While this does activate motor units and supports proprioceptive input, the absence of repetitive isometric contraction-relax cycles means that the total motor unit recruitment may be less extensive compared to PNF. Furthermore, the lack of a distinct relaxation phase following isometric tension may limit the effectiveness of Golgi tendon organ, thereby reducing the short-term neuromuscular window in which deeper flexibility gains can be realized. While Mulligan BLR still contributes meaningfully to joint mobilization and muscle elongation, its mechanical emphasis on joint correction and positional realignment may not be as effective in targeting deep muscle fiber recruitment and neuromuscular remodeling, especially when rapid flexibility improvements are required(Kavith K, 2025).

The long-term implications of muscle activation patterns during stretching are significant. PNF's high contraction demand not only produces greater mechanical tension across muscle-tendon units but also facilitates structural adaptations such as increased sarcomeres in series, thereby improving extensibility at the myofibrillar level. These adaptations provide a biological foundation for sustained flexibility gains and may also contribute to better outcomes in populations with chronic muscle tightness or movement restrictions. Additionally, the repetitive and volitional nature of PNF stretching fosters motor learning, allowing the brain to reprogram its perception of end-range limits. As the central nervous system becomes accustomed to greater ROMs where resetting the muscle's neural thresholds which effectively improves the movement efficiency and reducing the risk of re-injury (Sharman MJ, 2006). Mulligan BLR, although active and proprioceptively rich, does not emphasize the same level of contraction-relax repetition, which may explain the comparatively lower neuromuscular adaptations observed in the current study.

Beyond flexibility alone, PNF also contributes to strength maintenance and injury prevention, as it promotes functional lengthening without compromising muscle tension integrity. By engaging a broader spectrum of motor units, including those involved in force generation and stabilization, PNF enables individuals to maintain strength across the new ROM, an essential factor in avoiding joint instability or hypermobility-related injuries. Mulligan BLR, while beneficial for restoring positional faults and facilitating functional movement patterns, may not deliver the same strength-preserving benefits, especially if used in isolation without additional neuromuscular strengthening components. In the context of the present trial, the larger effect sizes observed in ROM outcomes for the PNF group may thus be attributed not only to superior stretch-induced elongation but also to greater neural adaptation, enhanced motor unit recruitment, and deeper proprioceptive engagement. These mechanistic advantages support the preferential use of PNF Hold-Relax techniques when aiming for rapid, sustained, and performance-oriented flexibility gains, particularly in athletes, rehabilitation populations, and individuals recovering from movement-limiting musculoskeletal conditions(Konrad A, 2016).

4.6 Comparison with Existing Literature

The findings of this study correlate closely with and are supported by an expanding quantity of literature on examining the impacts of Proprioceptive Neuromuscular Facilitation and Mulligan Bent Leg Raise techniques on hamstring flexibility and muscular performance. Recent studies have confirmed the efficacy of both approaches; however, the PNF group demonstrated superior outcomes, particularly regarding range of motion, consistent with previous findings that highlight the distinct neuromuscular and proprioceptive mechanisms that contribute to PNF effectiveness.

For instance, Sumantri et al. (2023) reported that PNF stretching significantly improved hamstring flexibility (by 19.5%) in futsal athletes, far exceeding the gains achieved through static stretching (6.7%). The study attributed these gains to enhanced activation of autogenic and reciprocal inhibition mechanisms, which are foundational to the PNF method. Similarly, the current study demonstrated that participants who received PNF Hold-Relax (HR) intervention showed significantly greater improvements in ROM compared to those treated with the Mulligan BLR technique. This suggests that PNF's contract-relax method not only increases stretch tolerance but also produces more immediate and profound flexibility enhancements, potentially due to more extensive motor unit recruitment and neuromuscular control. Adding to this, Park et al. (2020) demonstrated that PNF stretching combined with low-intensity dynamic exercises produced more sustained improvements in flexibility than PNF alone. While the present study did not include a post-exercise dynamic component, the significant ROM gains observed in the PNF group underscore its standalone efficacy. These findings support the notion that neuromuscular facilitation techniques may have cumulative benefits when combined with other forms of movement, although even in isolation, PNF appears to outperform other strategies in flexibility outcomes.

The literature also supports the use of PNF in broader clinical contexts. For example, Alam et al. (2023) found that PNF stretching was significantly more effective than Muscle Energy Technique (MET) in improving hamstring flexibility and reducing pain in patients with knee osteoarthritis. This reinforces the idea that PNF's neuromuscular re-education and proprioceptive activation contribute not only to flexibility gains but also to improved joint function and pain modulation. These broader benefits may explain why, even in a population of healthy young adults, PNF led to both statistically and clinically superior ROM improvements in the current study.

Likewise, Reena et al. (2020) compared PNF Hold-Relax with passive stretching in young, active individuals and found that PNF produced significantly greater gains in hamstring flexibility, as measured by Back Saver Sit and Reach (BSSR) and Fingertip-to-Floor (FTF) tests. This parallels the present study's findings, where PNF demonstrated larger effect sizes in ROM improvement. The consistency between these findings further strengthens the argument for incorporating PNF into training and rehabilitation routines, especially for populations that demand rapid and reliable flexibility adaptations, such as athletes or post-injury patients. On the other hand, the literature continues to support Mulligan's BLR technique as a viable method for enhancing hamstring flexibility, particularly in cases of joint dysfunction or spinal mobility restrictions. Irfan et al. (2023) discovered that the combination of Mulligan BLR and static stretching markedly enhanced spine mobility and hamstring flexibility in individuals with nonspecific low back pain. The improvements were evaluated utilizing the Modified Schober Test and the Active Knee Extension Test, similar to the functional outcomes examined in the present trial. The Mulligan group in this study demonstrated statistically significant enhancements in both range of motion and muscle strength; however, these improvements were relatively less pronounced than those obtained through proprioceptive neuromuscular facilitation. This indicates that Mulligan BLR may be more suitable in clinical contexts where joint kinematics take preference over muscle extensibility.

Additional evidence from the broader field continues to confirm these trends. In a systematic review by Behm et al. (2021), PNF was found to be more effective than static stretching and other conventional methods in producing long-term improvements in flexibility without compromising strength, especially in active populations. This supports the current study's observation that while both PNF and Mulligan BLR improve hamstring performance, PNF produces greater flexibility gains without a trade-off in muscle strength. Similarly, Konrad et al. (2021) found that PNF stretching leads to greater reductions in passive muscle stiffness and more sustainable flexibility increases than static stretching, attributing these effects to changes in viscoelastic properties and neuromuscular inhibition helps further validate the mechanisms proposed in the present study.

In contrast, although Mulligan techniques have shown strong clinical value, their mode of action is primarily based on joint mobilization and pain-free repositioning, rather than targeted neuromuscular activation. As a result, while they can effectively restore movement in conditions like NSLBP or postural misalignment, they may not produce the same level of muscular adaptation or cortical reprogramming as observed with PNF. The current findings are consistent with this distinction: while Mulligan BLR improved flexibility and strength, its effect size was smaller compared to PNF, particularly in terms of ROM outcomes. This indicates that PNF may be more suitable when addressing muscle-dominant flexibility restrictions, whereas Mulligan BLR may be ideal for joint-centric dysfunctions where alignment, accessory motion, or joint capsule mobility is limited.

Collectively, the present study contributes to the existing literature by directly comparing these two manual therapy interventions in a single experimental design, a comparison that is not extensively explored in current research. The results not only reaffirm the documented benefits of PNF for improving flexibility and muscular performance but also support the use of Mulligan BLR as a viable, though slightly less potent, alternative. This comparison is especially valuable for clinicians aiming to match treatment strategies to patient-specific needs such as favoring PNF for maximizing range of motion or using Mulligan BLR when joint repositioning or patient tolerance is a priority.

In conclusion, the present study's outcomes are in strong relation with recent research that supports the clinical value of both PNF and Mulligan BLR interventions. However, by demonstrating significantly greater improvements in hamstring ROM and slightly higher (though not statistically significant) strength gains in the PNF group, this study strengthens the argument for using PNF as the preferred technique when rapid and substantial flexibility enhancement is the clinical goal. The integration of current evidence with these findings underscores the relevance of PNF in both athletic and rehabilitation settings, while also reinforcing the practical utility of Mulligan techniques where patient comfort, joint mobilization, or passive correction is indicated.

4.7 Strengths of the Study in Clinical Application

The primary strength of the current study is its direct clinical applicability, providing physiotherapists and rehabilitation professionals with clear, evidence-based insights into the effectiveness of two widely used manual therapy techniques Proprioceptive Neuromuscular Facilitation (PNF) Hold-Relax and Mulligan Bent Leg Raise (BLR) in improving hamstring flexibility and muscle performance. While numerous studies have investigated these techniques independently, this study stands out by offering a direct head-to-head comparison, conducted under a controlled and standardized protocol. This design not only enhances the internal validity of the findings but also makes the results readily translatable to clinical practice, where therapists often need to decide between multiple interventions based on patient goals, tolerance, and resource availability.

From a clinical perspective, the findings offer valuable guidance for treatment selection. The statistically and clinically significant improvements in hamstring range of motion (ROM) and muscle strength observed in both intervention groups affirm the utility of both PNF and Mulligan BLR as effective, evidence-based tools for managing hamstring tightness and movement dysfunction. However, the greater ROM gains recorded in the PNF group, supported by very large effect sizes, offer a compelling case for its use when rapid improvements in flexibility are desired such as in athletic populations, post-operative cases requiring early mobilization, or patients with high functional demands. The evidence generated by this study enables clinicians to make more targeted and outcome-oriented decisions, choosing PNF when neuromuscular facilitation and motor learning are central goals, and Mulligan BLR when joint repositioning or spinal alignment is a contributing factor to hamstring dysfunction(Mishra A, 2024).

A significant advantage of this study is its emphasis on healthy young individuals, a population frequently engaged in physical activity or sports, where tight hamstrings are common and may contribute to movement inefficiency or injury. By selecting this group, the study reflects the real-world scenarios faced by physiotherapists working in sports clinics, orthopedic outpatient settings, and university wellness programs. This enhances the applicability of the findings, as most active adults seeking physiotherapy therapies often belong to a similar demographic group. Furthermore, the homogeneity of the sample (in terms of age, BMI, and activity level) controlled for potential confounders, thereby enhancing the internal consistency of the intervention effects. This methodological clarity ensures that the improvements observed were most likely due to the interventions themselves rather than baseline variability among participants(Akhtar H, 2023).

Clinically, the study's protocol was simple, reproducible, and reflective of routine physiotherapy practice. Both interventions were delivered in a single session and the outcome measures range of motion (ROM) and muscle strength were chosen because they are objective, clinically relevant, and commonly used in practice. The use of tools such as goniometry and dynamometry for measurement enhances the reliability and clinical utility of the findings, allowing therapists to adopt similar assessment techniques in their settings. This simplicity strengthens the external validity of the study and promotes ease of implementation in real-world practice, without requiring specialized equipment or lengthy training in complex procedures(Lopez N, 2018).

Additionally, the study emphasized both flexibility and muscle performance, acknowledging the importance of preserving or enhancing strength during stretching interventions. This dual-outcome approach is particularly relevant in sports and rehabilitation, where the risk of over-lengthening muscles leads to reduced force generation and this must be balanced against the need for improved range. The finding that PNF produced superior flexibility gains without compromising strength has significant implications for injury prevention strategies. It assures clinicians that using PNF Hold-Relax not only enhances extensibility but also maintains the functional integrity of the muscle, making it a safe and performance-enhancing option in diverse populations.

Finally, the findings contribute to a broader paradigm shift in physiotherapy from passive modalities to active and patient-engaged techniques. Both PNF and Mulligan BLR involve patient participation, which is essential for motor learning, proprioceptive feedback, and long-term retention of movement patterns. By validating the effectiveness of these active approaches, the study aligns with modern rehabilitation principles that emphasize patient empowerment, functional training, and the integration of neuromuscular systems for sustainable improvement. This alignment further enhances the clinical relevance of the research and supports the implementation of these methods in contemporary physiotherapy models(Schoeb V, 2011).

In summary, this study demonstrates several strengths from a clinical application standpoint. It offers a methodologically rigorous, directly applicable, and clinically relevant comparison of two widely used manual therapy techniques. The clarity of its intervention protocols, the objectivity of its outcome measures, the applicability to real-world patient populations, and the integration of neuromuscular and biomechanical perspectives all combine to make the findings highly valuable for physiotherapists seeking effective strategies to enhance flexibility, preserve strength, and promote functional movement. These strengths not only elevate the scientific contribution of the study but also provide immediate, actionable insights for clinical practice across sports, orthopedics, and rehabilitation domains.

4.8 Limitations of the Study

This study provides significant clinical insights and contributes to the comparative literature on manual therapy interventions for hamstring tightness; nevertheless, many limitations must be recognized to better understand the findings and guidance in future research direction.

A primary strength of this study is that outcome measurements were taken after three follow-up intervention sessions which strengthens the reliability of the findings by reflecting short-term treatment effectiveness rather than immediate, potentially transient, changes. However, despite this improvement over single-session designs, the study remains limited by the absence of a long-term follow-up phase. No data were collected beyond the third session to assess whether the observed improvements in hamstring range of motion (ROM) and muscle strength were retained over time. Flexibility gains achieved through neuromuscular adaptations or changes in stretch tolerance may regress without continued maintenance or self-directed exercises. Therefore, while the improvements captured after three sessions provide stronger evidence of intervention efficacy than immediate post-treatment measures, the long-term sustainability of these gains remains unknown. Including follow-ups at intervals such as one month or three months would allow for the assessment of retention and decay rates of flexibility and strength improvements.

Another limitation lies in the homogeneity of the sample, which comprised healthy young adults. This population was appropriate for controlling confounding variables and targeting early intervention strategies. However, it also restricts the generalizability of the findings to clinical populations such as older adults, sedentary individuals, or patients with neurological impairments. These groups may respond differently due to variations in tissue elasticity, proprioception, joint health, or neuromuscular control. Consequently, although the results are significantly relevant to physically active persons, prudence is required when attempting to generalize the findings to more intricate or pathologically varied populations.

Additionally, muscle strength was measured using a handheld dynamometer which is a relatively objective and practical tool in clinical research. The results may still be influenced by participant effort, fatigue, or learning effects. Isometric strength testing is inherently effort-dependent, and while standardization was enforced through consistent instructions and positioning, variability in maximal voluntary contraction may introduce minor inconsistencies. Moreover, the study lacked complementary neuromuscular assessments such as surface electromyography (sEMG), which could have provided a more detailed picture of motor unit recruitment and activation dynamics. Including EMG analysis in future studies would help verify whether PNF truly recruits more motor units or facilitates superior neuromuscular coordination compared to Mulligan BLR.

The single-blind design is another consideration. Although the assessor who performed the measurements was blinded to group allocation, the participants were aware of the intervention they received. This could introduce performance or expectation bias, especially if participants had preconceptions about one method being more effective than the other. For example, the interactive nature of PNF (involving resisted isometric contractions) may have given participants the perception of a more "active" or "intense" treatment, influencing their perceived outcomes or effort levels. While blinding participants in manual therapy studies is inherently challenging, the influence of participant expectations remains a potential confounding variable(Shmidt E, 2022).

Furthermore, the study did not account for participants' baseline physical activity levels, flexibility routines, or history of stretching interventions. These factors could act as effect modifiers, influencing how individuals respond to a particular technique. For example, an athlete accustomed to regular dynamic stretching may respond differently to PNF than a sedentary individual with low stretch tolerance. The absence of stratification or adjustment for these variables may have introduced variability in responsiveness, even though demographic and anthropometric data were relatively homogeneous.

In terms of clinical outcome measures, the study focused exclusively on ROM and isometric strength, which are important but represent only part of the functional picture. Incorporating functional performance assessments such as gait analysis, vertical jump height, or time-to-complete functional mobility tasks would help determine whether the observed physiological improvements translate into meaningful real-world benefits. This is particularly relevant in sports and rehabilitation contexts, where functional capacity, coordination, and movement efficiency are the ultimate goals of treatment.

The study also lacked mechanistic exploration through imaging, neurophysiological, or biomechanical analysis. While theoretical mechanisms such as reciprocal inhibition, Golgi tendon organ activation, and joint mobilization were discussed, no direct measurements were taken to validate these mechanisms in practice. Future research incorporating modalities like ultrasound elastography, motion analysis, or functional MRI could provide deeper insight into the specific physiological and neurological pathways activated by each intervention.

In conclusion, while this study addressed several methodological limitations common in manual therapy research such as improving measurement reliability through follow-ups and using objective testing tools it is still constrained by the absence of long-term follow-up, the limited generalizability to diverse populations, the lack of functional outcome measures, and the inability to explore underlying mechanisms directly. Future studies should incorporate larger, more diverse samples including functional and neurophysiological assessments, and evaluate the durability of intervention effects over time to further strengthen the evidence base for these widely used physiotherapy techniques.

4.9 Suggestions for Future Research

This study provides significant insights into the comparative effectiveness of the Proprioceptive Neuromuscular Facilitation Hold-Relax and Mulligan Bent Leg Raise approaches for enhancing hamstring flexibility and muscle strength, while also suggesting multiple directions for further research. Future research might enhance the understanding of these therapies by targeting several critical areas while considering the findings and understanding the methodological limitations.

One of the most critical recommendations is the incorporation of long-term follow-up assessments. While this study evaluated outcomes after three treatment sessions, it remains unclear whether the gains in range of motion and muscle strength are maintained over extended periods. Future research should include follow-up evaluations at 1 month, 3 months, and possibly even 6 months post-intervention to assess the retention of flexibility improvements and strength adaptations. Longitudinal data would help determine whether either technique leads to more sustainable outcomes, which is essential for guiding treatment plans and advising patients on the need for maintenance programs(Cuzick J, 2022).

Another priority for future research is the inclusion of more diverse populations, particularly clinical groups that are commonly affected by hamstring tightness and musculoskeletal dysfunction. These might include older adults, sedentary individuals, patients recovering from lower limb injuries, individuals with neurological conditions such as stroke or multiple sclerosis or those experiencing chronic conditions such as low back pain or osteoarthritis. Studying these populations would provide more generalizable evidence regarding the safety, feasibility, and effectiveness of PNF and Mulligan techniques across varying physical, neurological, and biomechanical profiles.

Moreover, future studies should consider integrating functional outcome measures in addition to physiological metrics such as ROM and strength. While these variables are valuable and frequently used in clinical practice, they do not fully capture how improvements translate into real-life performance. Including tests like the Functional Movement Screen (FMS), Timed Up and Go (TUG), sit-to-stand tests, gait analysis, or athletic performance measures such as sprint times or vertical jump height would allow researchers to assess whether manual therapy interventions improve functional capacity and movement quality in ways that are meaningful to daily life, sports performance, and rehabilitation goals(Lim JH, 2023).

To further explore the mechanisms underlying treatment effects, future research should adopt a multi-modal assessment approach. The addition of surface electromyography (sEMG), ultrasound elastography, joint stiffness measurements, or even functional neuroimaging could help clarify how these interventions influence neuromuscular recruitment, tendon and fascia behavior, and central nervous system adaptation. For example, EMG could reveal whether PNF leads to greater activation of both slow- and fast-twitch motor units, supporting the hypothesis of superior muscle fiber engagement. Likewise, elastography could provide real-time insights into changes in muscle or fascia stiffness before and after each intervention, offering concrete physiological evidence for the proposed mechanisms of elongation and inhibition.

An opportunity exists to investigate the dose-response correlation of both PNF and Mulligan BLR methods. Future research may adjust variables including repetition count, contraction intensity, hold time, hip flexion angle, and session frequency to determine ideal procedures. This will bolster evidence-based therapeutic guidelines for customizing therapies to the distinct requirements of diverse patient populations, including athletes, post-operative persons, or those with elevated muscle tone. Comparisons across various PNF procedures, such as Hold-Relax, Contract-Relax, Agonist Contraction, and Mulligan variations, could provide valuable insights into which specific methods produce the most beneficial results under distinct scenarios.

Additionally, future research could investigate the psychological and perceptual dimensions of stretching interventions. Variables such as perceived comfort, stretch tolerance, sense of control, and treatment satisfaction may influence patient compliance and clinical outcomes. Including validated questionnaires or patient-reported outcome measures (PROMs) could offer a more holistic understanding of how patients experience these interventions and whether those perceptions impact effectiveness. This is especially relevant in modern rehabilitation, where patient-centered care and shared decision-making are becoming increasingly prioritized(Russo-Netzer P, 2022).

Comparative studies could also be extended to include other manual therapy techniques, such as Instrument-Assisted Soft Tissue Mobilization (IASTM), Myofascial Release (MFR), or Muscle Energy Technique (MET), to position PNF and Mulligan BLR within a broader therapeutic context. These comparisons would help physiotherapists make more informed decisions based on factors such as clinical goals, time constraints, equipment availability, and patient preference. Moreover, studies comparing manual vs. self-stretching protocols or examining the combined effect of manual therapy and exercise-based rehabilitation could help establish multi-modal approaches that yield synergistic benefits. Another valuable direction is the evaluation of these interventions in telerehabilitation or home-based formats, especially in light of the increasing demand for remote therapy options. Investigating whether techniques like PNF or simplified Mulligan movements can be delivered effectively through video consultation would help expand accessibility, especially for patients in rural areas or those with mobility limitations.

Lastly, future work could aim to explore educational strategies for improving therapist competency in delivering these interventions. Investigating the impact of therapist experience, training quality, or technique standardization on clinical outcomes could help develop training curricula, ensuring that manual therapy techniques like PNF and Mulligan are delivered consistently and effectively in both academic and clinical settings.

Conclusion

This randomized controlled trial investigated and compared the efficacy of two manual therapy techniques—Proprioceptive Neuromuscular Facilitation (PNF) Hold-Relax and Mulligan Bent Leg Raise (BLR)—in enhancing hamstring flexibility and isometric muscle strength. Both interventions demonstrated statistically significant improvements in range of motion and strength. However, PNF Hold-Relax yielded superior gains in hamstring flexibility, evidenced by greater mean differences, stronger effect sizes, and higher statistical significance. These findings suggest that the neuromuscular activation and reflexive inhibition achieved through PNF promote more efficient elongation of muscle tissue compared to the mobilization-with-movement approach of Mulligan BLR. Despite this distinction in flexibility outcomes, muscle strength improvements were comparable between the groups, highlighting the potential of both techniques to preserve or enhance strength in the short term. This differentiation between interventions is clinically meaningful: PNF is particularly advantageous for achieving rapid improvements in flexibility, while Mulligan BLR remains useful for joint mobilization and movement correction, offering therapists options based on patient needs and treatment goals.

Clinically, these results underscore the value of selecting evidence-based techniques that align with rehabilitation objectives. Hamstring tightness contributes to postural issues, gait dysfunction, and injury risk across both athletic and sedentary populations, making its management a cornerstone of physiotherapy. The superiority of PNF Hold-Relax in producing immediate gains positions it as a strong intervention in contexts demanding quick restoration of extensibility, such as sports performance or accelerated rehabilitation timelines. Mulligan BLR, with its gentler mobilization and dynamic application, may be preferred when prioritizing patient comfort or correcting movement patterns. Limitations of the study include its short-term scope, limited sample size, and lack of follow-up on long-term outcomes. Future research should expand on these findings by exploring durability of effects, integration with complementary interventions such as strength or proprioceptive training, and underlying neuromechanical or cortical mechanisms. By addressing these areas, future investigations can further refine physiotherapy practice and strengthen the evidence base guiding individualized, functionally driven rehabilitation.

References

Adnan M, Arsh A, Ali B, Ahmad S. Effectiveness of bent leg raise technique and neurodynamics in patients with radiating low back pain. Pakistan Journal of Medical Sciences. 2021 Nov 15;38(1).

1. Adnan M, Arsh A, Ali B, Ahmad S. Effectiveness of bent leg raise technique and neurodynamics in patients with radiating low back pain. Pakistan Journal of Medical Sciences. 2021 Nov 15;38(1).
2. Akhtar H, Muskan P, Amjad R, Satti AK, Javed M, Shahid M. Correlation of Hamstring Tightness with Balance and Mobility in Young Adults. Pakistan Journal of Medical and Health Sciences. 2023 Apr 20;17(3):295–7.
3. Alexandre de Assis IS, Luvizutto GJ, Bruno ACM, Sande de Souza LAP. The Proprioceptive Neuromuscular Facilitation Concept in Parkinson Disease: A Systematic Review and Meta-Analysis. Journal of Chiropractic Medicine [Internet]. 2020 Sep;19(3):181–7. Available from:
4. Aye T, Kuramoto-Ahuja T, Han H, Maruyama H. Comparison of immediate effects between two medical stretching techniques on Hamstrings flexibility. Journal of Physical Therapy Science. 2017;29(9):1518–21.
5. Bharat Masekar M, Rayjade DrA, Yadav DrTrupti, Chotai DrKhushboo. Effectiveness of Muscle Energy Technique and Proprioceptive Neuromuscular Facilitation in Knee Osteoarthritis. International Journal of pharma and Bio Sciences. 2021 Jan 23;11(1):16–22.

6. Blackburn JT, Norcross MF, Cannon LN, Zinder SM. Hamstrings Stiffness and Landing Biomechanics Linked to Anterior Cruciate Ligament Loading. Journal of Athletic Training [Internet]. 2013 Dec;48(6):764–72. Available from:
7. Bonnar BP, Deivert RG, Gould TE. The relationship between isometric contraction durations during hold-relax stretching and improvement of hamstring flexibility. The Journal of Sports Medicine and Physical Fitness [Internet]. 2004 Sep 1 [cited 2022 May 12];44(3):258–61. Available from:
8. Buckthorpe M, Wright S, Bruce-Low S, Nanni G, Sturdy T, Gross AS, et al. Recommendations for hamstring injury prevention in elite football: translating research into practice. British Journal of Sports Medicine [Internet]. 2018 Nov 9;53(7):449–56. Available from:
9. Chu SK, Rho ME. Hamstring injuries in the athlete. Current Sports Medicine Reports [Internet]. 2016;15(3):184–90. Available from:
10. Claudino JG, Cardoso Filho CA, Bittencourt NFN, Gonçalves LG, Couto CR, Quintão RC, et al. Eccentric Strength Assessment of Hamstring Muscles with New Technologies: a Systematic Review of Current Methods and Clinical Implications. Sports Medicine - Open [Internet]. 2021 Jan 28;7(1).
11. Croisier JL, Ganteaume S, Binet J, Genty M, Ferret JM. Strength Imbalances and Prevention of Hamstring Injury in Professional Soccer Players. The American Journal of Sports Medicine. 2008 Aug;36(8):1469–75.
12. Cuzick J. The importance of long-term follow up of participants in clinical trials. British Journal of Cancer. 2022 Dec 1;128(1):432–8.
13. Comparison Between Straight Leg Raise and Bent Leg Raise Stretching Techniques for Increasing Hamstring Flexibility in Healthy Male Volunteers. *Int J Creative Sci Publ* [Internet]. 2024 [cited 2025 Sep 24];2(4):327-332. Available from: https://rjpn.org/ijcspub/papers/IJCSP24B1327.pdf
14. de Sire A, Marotta N, Spanó R, Fasano S, Sgro M, Lippi L, et al. Efficacy of proprioceptive neuromuscular facilitation on functioning in patients with bilateral hip osteoarthritis: A pilot randomized controlled trial. Journal of Back and Musculoskeletal Rehabilitation [Internet]. 2024 Jan 1;37(2):445–57. Available from:

15. Decoster LC, Cleland J, Altieri C. The Effects of Hamstring Stretching on Range of Motion: A Systematic Literature Review. Journal of Orthopaedic & Sports Physical Therapy. 2005 Jun;35(6):377–87.
16. Encarnación-Martínez A, García-Gallart A, Pérez-Soriano P, Catalá-Vilaplana I, Rizo-Albero J, Sanchis-Sanchis R. Effect of Hamstring Tightness and Fatigue on Dynamic Stability and Agility in Physically Active Young Men. Sensors [Internet]. 2023 Jan 1;23(3):1633. Available from:
17. Encarnación-Martínez A, García-Gallart A, Pérez-Soriano P, Catalá-Vilaplana I, Rizo-Albero J, Sanchis-Sanchis R. Effect of Hamstring Tightness and Fatigue on Dynamic Stability and Agility in Physically Active Young Men. Sensors [Internet]. 2023 Jan 1;23(3):1633. Available from:
18. ElMeligie MM, Abdeen HA, Atef H, Marques-Sule E, Karkosha RN. The effectiveness of mulligan mobilization with movement (MWM) on outcomes of patients with ankle sprain: a systematic review and meta-analysis. BMC Sports Science, Medicine and Rehabilitation [Internet]. 2025 Apr 29;17(1). Available from: https://pmc.ncbi.nlm.nih.gov/articles/PMC12042638/
19. Gaku Tokutake, Rieko Kuramochi, Murata Y, Shota Enoki, Koto Y, Shimizu T. The Risk Factors of Hamstring Strain Injury Induced by High-Speed Running. Journal of Sports Science & Medicine [Internet]. 2018 Nov 20;17(4):650. Available from:
20. Gou Y, Lei H, Chen X, Wang X. The effects of hamstring stretching exercises on pain intensity and function in low back pain patients: A systematic review with meta-analysis of randomized controlled trials. SAGE Open Medicine [Internet]. 2024 Jan 1;12. Available from: https://www.ncbi.nlm.nih.gov/pmc/articles/PMC11289822/
21. Haab T, Wydra G. The effect of age on hamstring passive properties after a 10-week stretch training. Journal of Physical Therapy Science. 2017;29(6):1048–53.
22. Hall T, Hardt S, Schäfer A, Wallin L. Mulligan bent leg raise technique—a preliminary randomized trial of immediate effects after a single intervention. Manual Therapy. 2006 May;11(2):130–5.
23. Hindle K, Whitcomb T, Briggs W, Hong J. Proprioceptive Neuromuscular Facilitation (PNF): Its Mechanisms and Effects on Range of Motion and Muscular Function. Journal of Human Kinetics [Internet]. 2012 Mar 1;31(1):105–13. Available from:

24. Hussein H, Atteya M, Ansari A, Kamel E. A Systematic Review and Meta-Analysis of the Effectiveness of Mulligan Mobilization with Movement on Pain, Range of Motion, Function, and Flexibility in Patients with Sciatica. Neurorehabilitation. 2024 Dec 18;
25. Irfan A, Mannan R, Aleena, Riaz S, Rashid S, Khan RR. Effects of Mulligan's Bent Leg Raise Technique on Hamstring Flexibility and Lumbar Spine Mobility in Healthy Females. Pakistan Journal of Medical and Health Sciences. 2023 Jan 31;17(1):407–9.
26. Jandre Reis FJ, Macedo AR. Influence of Hamstring Tightness in Pelvic, Lumbar and Trunk Range of Motion in Low Back Pain and Asymptomatic Volunteers during Forward Bending. Asian Spine Journal [Internet]. 2015;9(4):535. Available from:
27. Kavith K, Nandhini M. Effectiveness of Various Mulligan Techniques on Hamstring Flexibility in College Level Cricketers. 2023 [cited 2025 Apr 4];5. Available from:
28. Kaya M, Hikmet Ucgun, Hilal Denizoglu Kulli. The effect of proprioceptive neuromuscular facilitation on individuals with text neck syndrome: A randomized controlled study. Medicine [Internet]. 2024 Jul 26 [cited 2024 Oct 23];103(30):e38716–6. Available from:
29. Kim G, Kim H, Kim WK, Kim J. Effect of stretching-based rehabilitation on pain, flexibility and muscle strength in dancers with hamstring injury: a single-blind, prospective, randomized clinical trial. The Journal of Sports Medicine and Physical Fitness [Internet]. 2018 Sep 1;58(9):1287–95. Available from:
30. Konrad A, Stafilidis S, Tilp M. Effects of acute static, ballistic, and PNF stretching exercise on the muscle and tendon tissue properties. Scandinavian Journal of Medicine & Science in Sports [Internet]. 2016 Jul 1;27(10):1070–80. Available from:
31. KS S, Heggannavar A, Metgud S. The effect of Mulligan's Bent Leg Raise versus Instrument Assisted Soft Tissue Mobilization in subjects with hamstring tightness in non-specific low backache: A randomized clinical trial. International Journal of Physiotherapy. 2019 Aug 1;6(4).
32. Kumar N, Kumar S, None Prathap Suganthirababu, None Jagatheesan Alagesan. Effectiveness of Pnf Stretching in Hamstring Tightness Population Having Low Back Pain. Indian Journal of Physiotherapy and Occupational Therapy. 2024 Jan 21;18:651–6.

33. Lim JH, Kim SY, Kim BG. A Survey on the Use of Outcome Measures during Physical Therapy Interventions by Physical Therapists in Korea. Healthcare. 2023 Nov 9;11(22):2933–3.
34. Kosova A, Pala OO. Does Proprioceptive Neuromuscular Facilitation-Based Hamstring Stretching Influence Deep Cervical Flexor Muscle Endurance? Life. 2025 Jun 26;15(7):1019.
35. Liyanage E, Kavinda Malwanage, Dilhari Senarath, Hashini Wijayasinghe, Indrajith Liyanage, Dhananjee Chellapillai, et al. Effects of Different Physical Therapy Interventions in Improving Flexibility in University Students with Hamstring Tightness - A Systematic Review and Network Meta-analysis. International Journal of Exercise Science [Internet]. 2024 Mar;17(3):359. Available from:
36. Lopez N, Perez E, Tello E, Rodrigo A, Valentinuzzi ME. Statistical Validation for Clinical Measures: Repeatability and Agreement of KinectTM-Based Software. BioMed Research International. 2018;2018:1–11.
37. López-Miñarro P, Muyor J, Belmonte F, Alacid F. Accepted for printing in. Journal of Human Kinetics [Internet]. 2012;31:69–78. Available from:
38. Madhubabu Kothapalli. Influence of prolonged sitting time on development of hamstring muscle tightness in desk job employees. Health, Sport & Rehabilitation Medicine. 2023 Dec 15;24(4):182–5.
39. Manabendra Majhi, Mondal S, Chatterjee S. Understanding the theoretical mechanisms behind proprioceptive neuromuscular facilitation through the experimental studies on brain. Indian Journal Of Applied Research [Internet]. 2021 Jun 30;11(03):89–94. Available from:
40. Maniar N, Carmichael DS, Hickey JT, Timmins RG, San Jose AJ, Dickson J, et al. Incidence and prevalence of hamstring injuries in field-based team sports: a systematic review and meta-analysis of 5952 injuries from over 7 million exposure hours. British Journal of Sports Medicine. 2022 Dec 1;57(2):bjsports-2021-104936.
41. Marek SM, Cramer JT, Fincher AL, Massey LL, Dangelmaier SM, Sushmita Purkayastha, et al. Acute Effects of Static and Proprioceptive Neuromuscular Facilitation Stretching on Muscle Strength and Power Output. Journal of Athletic Training [Internet]. 2025;40(2):94. Available from:

42. Mateos-Aparicio P, Rodríguez-Moreno A. The impact of studying Brain Plasticity. Frontiers in Cellular Neuroscience. 2019;13(66).

43. Mishra A, Sharvani B. Comparison of proprioceptive neuro-muscular facilitation and mulligan stretching on hamstring tightness in recreational football players. International Journal of Physical Education, Sports and Health [Internet]. 2024 Jul 1 [cited 2025 Apr 4];11(4):323–7. Available from:

44. Muyor JM, López-Miñarro PA, Casimiro AJ. Effect of stretching program in an industrial workplace on hamstring flexibility and sagittal spinal posture of adult women workers: A randomized controlled trial. Journal of Back and Musculoskeletal Rehabilitation. 2012 Aug 20;25(3):161–9.

45. Oleksy Ł, Mika A, Pacana J, Markowska O, Stolarczyk A, Kielnar R. Why Is Hamstring Strain Injury so Common in Sport Despite Numerous Prevention Methods? Are There Any Missing Pieces to This Puzzle? Frontiers in Physiology. 2021 May 13;12.

46. Opar DA, Williams MD, Shield AJ. Hamstring Strain Injuries. Sports Medicine. 2012 Mar;42(3):209–26.

47. P. M, K.kavith, M. Nandhini. Effectiveness of Various Mulligan Techniques on Hamstring Flexibility in College Level Cricketers. International Journal For Multidisciplinary Research. 2023 Aug 20;5(4).

48. PAGEPress. Stretching exercises in managing spasticity: effectiveness, risks, and adjunct therapies | European Journal of Translational Myology [Internet]. Pagepressjournals.org. 2023 [cited 2025 Apr 4]. Available from:

49. Park S, Lim W. Effects of Proprioceptive Neuromuscular Facilitation Stretching at Low-intensities with Standing Toe Touch on Developing and Maintaining Hamstring Flexibility. Journal of Bodywork and Movement Therapies. 2020 Sep;

50. Patel P, Shukla M. Relationship between Sitting Hours, Physical Activity and Hamstring Flexibility. 2023 Jan 18 [cited 2025 Mar 28];24–9. Available from:

51. Pourahmadi M, Sahebalam M, Bagheri R. Effectiveness of Proprioceptive Neuromuscular Facilitation on Pain Intensity and Functional Disability in Patients with Low Back Pain: A Systematic Review and Meta-Analysis. The Archives of Bone and Joint Surgery [Internet]. 2020 Jul [cited 2021 Aug 3];8(4):479–501. Available from:

52. Pratt J, Boreham C, Ennis S, Ryan AW, De Vito G. Genetic Associations with Aging Muscle: A Systematic Review. Cells [Internet]. 2019 Dec 19 [cited 2020 Aug 14];9(1). Available from:
53. Prince C, Morin JB, Mendiguchia J, Lahti J, Guex K, Edouard P, et al. Sprint Specificity of Isolated Hamstring-Strengthening Exercises in Terms of Muscle Activity and Force Production. Frontiers in Sports and Active Living. 2021 Jan 21;2.
54. R R, Paul J, Kumar P. To compare the effectiveness of passive stretching versus PNF hold relax technique on hamstring tightness in young individuals. International Journal Medical and Exercise Science. 2020 Mar 17;06(01):668–75.
55. Rahul Krishnan Kutty, Ong Sıew Chee, Suvınlal Stalın, Dewan S. A comparative analysis of various proprioceptive neuromuscular facilitation (PNF) techniques on muscle flexibility among extended sitting posture individuals. Türk fizyoterapi ve rehabilitasyon dergisi [Internet]. 2023 Jun 1 [cited 2024 Aug 27]; Available from:
56. Ramos GA, Arliani GG, Astur DC, Pochini A de C, Ejnisman B, Cohen M. Rehabilitation of hamstring muscle injuries: a literature review. Revista Brasileira de Ortopedia (English Edition) [Internet]. 2017 Jan;52(1):11–6. Available from:
57. Reiner M, Tilp M, Guilhem G, Morales-Artacho A, Nakamura M, Konrad A. Effects of a Single Proprioceptive Neuromuscular Facilitation Stretching Exercise With and Without Post-stretching Activation on the Muscle Function and Mechanical Properties of the Plantar Flexor Muscles. Frontiers in Physiology. 2021 Sep 14;12.
58. Rodgers CD, Raja A. Anatomy, Bony Pelvis and Lower Limb, Hamstring Muscle [Internet]. PubMed. Treasure Island (FL): StatPearls Publishing; 2023. Available from:
59. Russo-Netzer P, Cohen GL. “If you’re uncomfortable, go outside your comfort zone”: A novel behavioral “stretch” intervention supports the well-being of unhappy people. The Journal of Positive Psychology. 2022 May 15;18(3):1–17.
60. Schoeb V, Bürge E. Perceptions of Patients and Physiotherapists on Patient Participation: A Narrative Synthesis of Qualitative Studies. Physiotherapy Research International [Internet]. 2011 Jul 13;17(2):80–91. Available from:
61. Senduran Yıldırım M, Ozyürek S, Celiker Tosun O, Uzer S, Gelecek N. Comparison of effects of static, proprioceptive neuromuscular facilitation and Mulligan stretching on hip

flexion range of motion: a randomized controlled trial. Biology of Sport. 2016 Jan 1;33(1):89–94.

62. Sharman MJ, Cresswell AG, Riek S. Proprioceptive Neuromuscular Facilitation Stretching. Sports Medicine [Internet]. 2006;36(11):929–39. Available from:
63. Shimura K, Kasai T. Effects of proprioceptive neuromuscular facilitation on the initiation of voluntary movement and motor evoked potentials in upper limb muscles. Human Movement Science [Internet]. 2002 [cited 2025 Apr 3];21:101–13. Available from:
64. Shmidt E, Jacobson BC. Double-Blind Reviews. Clinical and Translational Gastroenterology. 2022 Jan 11;Publish Ahead of Print.
65. Sita A. The effectivity of back massage with Mulligan Bent Leg Raise in ultrasound intervention to reduce pain and disability in mechanical low back pain [Internet]. Jurnal Harian Regional. 2021 [cited 2025 Apr 1]. Available from:
66. Sivasubramaniyan K, Arul Pragassame S, Srinivasan B, Jerry C, Pragassame S. Effect of Mulligan Bent Leg Raise Technique on Low Back Pain Subjects with Radiculopathy. 2022 [cited 2024 May 24];21. Available from:
67. Smedes F, Giacometti da Silva L. Motor learning with the PNF-concept, an alternative to constrained induced movement therapy in a patient after a stroke; a case report. Journal of Bodywork and Movement Therapies [Internet]. 2019 Jul 1 [cited 2020 Feb 22];23(3):622–7. Available from:
68. Spernoga SG, Uhl TL, Arnold BL, Gansneder BM. Duration of Maintained Hamstring Flexibility After a One-Time, Modified Hold-Relax Stretching Protocol. Journal of Athletic Training [Internet]. 2025 [cited 2025 Mar 31];36(1):44. Available from:
69. Spinoso DH, Goulart M, Ferreira A, Navega M. Analysis of the relationship between hamstring flexibility with muscular strength and its response to myofascial release. Manual Therapy, Posturology & Rehabilitation Journal. 2022 Sep 15;20:1–7.
70. Stathopoulos N, Dimitriadis Z, Koumantakis GA. Effectiveness of Mulligan's mobilization with movement techniques on pain and disability of peripheral joints: a systematic review with meta-analysis between 2008–2017. Physiotherapy [Internet]. 2019 Mar [cited 2019 Nov 4];105(1):1–9. Available from:

71. Sugiura Y, Sakuma K, Sakuraba K, Sato Y. Prevention of Hamstring Injuries in Collegiate Sprinters. Orthopaedic Journal of Sports Medicine [Internet]. 2017 Jan;5(1):232596711668152. Available from:
72. Sumantri RJ, Soegiyanto, Rumini, Setyawati H, Suryadi D, Suganda MA. PNF stretching and static stretching exercises: Efforts to increase the flexibility of the hamstring muscles in futsal players [Internet]. Available from:
73. Sos-Tirado M, Aser Campo-Manzanares, Aguado-Oregui L, Carles Cerdá-Calatayud, Guardiola-Ruiz JC, García-Lucas C, et al. Short Term Effects of Proprioceptive Neuromuscular Facilitation Combined with Neuromuscular Electrical Stimulation in Youth Basketball Players: A Randomized Controlled Trial. Journal of Functional Morphology and Kinesiology. 2024 Dec 20;9(4):280–0.
74. Santosh Channabasapa Metgud, Patil SD, Omkar Anand Gaonkar. Immediate Effect of Kinetic Chain Activation and Mulligan's Bent Leg Raise Technique in Patients with Asymptomatic Hamstring Tightness: A Randomised Clinical Trial. Journal of Clinical and Diagnostic Research. 2025 Jan 1;
75. Theofanidis D, Fountouki A. Limitations and delimitations in the research process. Perioperative Nursing [Internet]. 2019;7(3):155–62. Available from:
76. Tomruk M, Tomruk MS, Gelecek N. Effects of Dynamic Extension Exercise and Mulligan Stretching on Hamstring Flexibility. Orthopaedic Journal of Sports Medicine [Internet]. 2014 Nov [cited 2019 Jun 21];2(11_suppl3):2325967114S0016. Available from:
77. Wan X, Li S, Best TM, Liu H, Li H, Yu B. Effects of flexibility and strength training on peak hamstring musculotendinous strains during sprinting. Journal of Sport and Health Science. 2020 Aug;10(2).
78. Wan X, Qu F, Garrett WE, Liu H, Yu B. Relationships among hamstring muscle optimal length and hamstring flexibility and strength. Journal of Sport and Health Science. 2017 Sep;6(3):275–82.
79. Wan X, Qu F, Garrett WE, Liu H, Yu B. The effect of hamstring flexibility on peak hamstring muscle strain in sprinting. Journal of Sport and Health Science. 2017 Sep 1;6(3):283–9.

80. Winter L, Huang Q, Sertic JVL, Konczak J. The Effectiveness of Proprioceptive Training for Improving Motor Performance and Motor Dysfunction: A Systematic Review. Frontiers in Rehabilitation Sciences. 2022 Apr 8;3.
81. Yadav R, Basista R. Effect of Prolonged Sitting on Hamstring Muscle Flexibility and Lumbar Lordosis in Collegiate Student. International Journal of Health Sciences and Research [Internet]. 2020 [cited 2023 Mar 30];10(9):280–9. Available from:
82. Youdas JW, Haeflinger KM, Kreun MK, Holloway AM, Kramer CM, Hollman JH. The efficacy of two modified proprioceptive neuromuscular facilitation stretching techniques in subjects with reduced hamstring muscle length. Physiotherapy Theory and Practice. 2010 Jan;26(4):240–50.

Publisher: Eliva Press Global Ltd

Email: info@elivapress.com

www.ingramcontent.com/pod-product-compliance
Lightning Source LLC
LaVergne TN
LVHW022311200926
848481LV00004B/1279